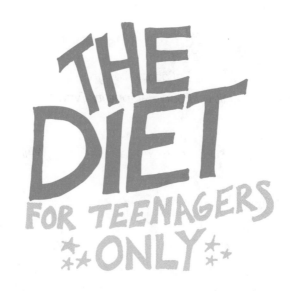

THE DIET
FOR TEENAGERS
★ ★ ONLY ★ ★

Also by Carrie Wiatt

Eating by Design:
The Individualized Food Personality Type Nutrition Plan

Portion Savvy:
The 30-Day Smart Plan for Eating Well

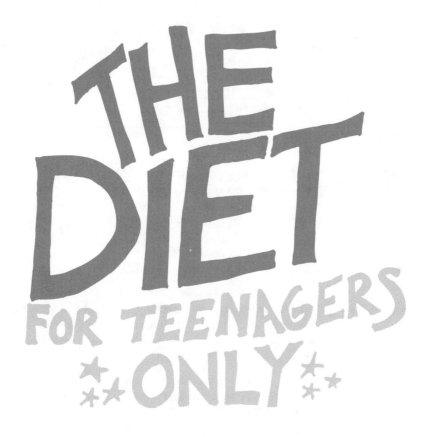

THE DIET
FOR TEENAGERS
★ ONLY ★

CARRIE WIATT AND
BARBARA SCHROEDER

HC

An Imprint of HarperCollinsPublishers

Photographs by Rachel Latt
Illustrations by Atousa Ziatabari

THE DIET FOR TEENAGERS ONLY. Copyright © 2005 by Carrie Wiatt and Barbara Schroeder. All rights reserved. Printed in the United States of America. No part of this book may be used or reproduced in any manner whatsoever without written permission except in the case of brief quotations embodied in critical articles and reviews. For information address HarperCollins Publishers Inc., 10 East 53rd Street, New York, NY 10022.

HarperCollins books may be purchased for educational, business, or sales promotional use. For information please write: Special Markets Department, HarperCollins Publishers Inc., 10 East 53rd Street, New York, NY 10022.

FIRST EDITION

Designed by Kris Tobiassen

Printed on acid-free paper

Library of Congress Cataloging-in-Publication Data

Wiatt, Carrie Latt.
    The diet for teenagers only / Carrie Wiatt & Barbara Schroeder.—1st ed.
        p. cm.
    ISBN 0-06-079361-9
    1. Teenage girls—Nutrition. 2. Teenage girls—Health and hygiene. 3. Eating disorders in adolescence—Prevention. 4. Reducing diets. 5. Diet. I. Schroeder, Barbara, 1958– II. Title.

RJ235.W53 2005
613.2'0835'2—dc22   2005042823

08 09 RRD 10

TO MY DAUGHTER, BELLA,
FOREVER IN MY HEART
          ☆ CARRIE WIATT

TO MY DARLING GLENN
AND DAUGHTERS EVERYWHERE
MAY YOU SEE YOUR BEAUTY
THE WAY YOUR MOMS DO!
          ☆ BARBARA SCHROEDER

CONTENTS

HELLO DARLING!

This book is for you. You're a teenager, and over 70 percent of teens are dissatisfied with their body or weight. That's a lot. Many of you might be on diets that are really designed for adults. Or you've already tried a bunch of different diets and ways to eat. (One girl we interviewed for this book said, "I ate a grape a meal. I figured that's what models do!")

Chances are, these dieting approaches aren't working for you for lots of reasons. They're hard to stick to. You're not really losing weight. And worst of all, you're probably hungry and feeling deprived a lot of the time. You might even feel guilty about the way you eat, and that doesn't feel good.

We want you to feel good about yourself! Which means you need special information, secret dieting tips, and most importantly, knowledge about what's happening to you and your body *right now.*

Here's the deal. You are in the biggest, most important growth spurt of your life. This is *the most critical* time for you to learn to eat right and treat your body with the respect (and the nutrition!) it *deserves.* If you don't, you might stunt your growth or develop health problems!

So that's why we got together. We want to give you the secrets to eating great and losing weight if you need to. Carrie runs an amazing business in Los Angeles called Diet Designs. She figures out how many calories, fat, and other nutrients each client needs (many of her clients are celebrities, including Melissa Joan Hart, Jewel, Salma Hayek, and Tiffani Amber Thiessen), then her company delivers fabulously delicious food to them. So not only does Carrie have a master's degree in nutrition, she also has real-life experience in designing diets that taste good and really help you lose weight. In this book, you'll find the best of Carrie's recipes and diet tips, specifically designed for teenagers only! (Wait until you try the Magic Muffin recipe!)

Barbara is an Emmy Award–winning reporter who has worked in Los Angeles for a long time and she has often interviewed Carrie on TV. Barbara also has a fifteen-year-old daughter, and they both have learned a lot about nutrition along the way.

So here's a diet designed *just for you* and your rapidly changing body. Follow it for 7 days and lose some weight. Then, if you need to lose more, you'll know how to do it safely and maintain your ideal weight for life. Our hope is that you'll never have difficult issues with food and weight again.

But be realistic. We want you to really, really understand that you should look the best you can for your body and body type. (Find out in chapter 3: Am I Fat?)

Don't forget, you have lots of pressure on you right now—school, boys, family stuff, friends, and popularity issues. Plus TV shows and magazines are flooding you with pictures of impossibly thin models!! You're also being bombarded by *thousands* of food ads a year, all trying to sway the way you eat. Don't let these images get to you!

Fight back, be as fit and nutritionally smart as you can be, and know that once you accept yourself and believe in yourself with all of your heart and soul, you'll be able to look in the mirror and say, "You know what, I like myself. Just the way I am!"

Let's get started!

Love,

Barbara and Carrie

DAUGHTER, I CANNOT GIVE YOU ANYTHING
SO COMPLETE OR PERFECT OR PURE. BUT I CAN
GIVE YOU SOMETHING BETTER. YOUR BODY . . .
AND THE FIERCE LOVE OF IT THAT NO ONE
CAN TAKE AWAY.

—LINDA NEMEC FOSTER,
FROM THE POEM "HISTORY OF THE BODY"
IN THE BOOK LIVING IN THE FIRE NEST

ONE **THINGS THEY NEVER TOLD YOU**

Grab a pen or pencil and take a few moments to write down, right here, what you think of your body and what you would change about it if you could do anything you wanted.

_____

_____

_____

_____

_____

_____

Here's what some of the girls who answered our teen diet surveys said:

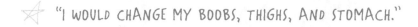 "I WOULD CHANGE MY BOOBS, THIGHS, AND STOMACH."

"I WOULD HAVE SKINNIER ARMS, A FLATTER TUMMY, AND NOT A CHUBBY CHIN."

"I'M THIRTEEN YEARS OF AGE. I WEIGH A MASSIVE 165 POUNDS. I'M SO SICK OF BEING FAT, BEING TEASED, AND NOT BEING ABLE TO FIT INTO ANY NICE, TRENDY CLOTHES. PLEASE HELP ME, SOMETIMES I FEEL LIKE I'M DROWNING."

"AT THE AGE OF NINETEEN, I'VE BEEN ON ABOUT TEN DIETS, AND I KEEP RE-GAINING THE WEIGHT I LOSE. HELP!"

Most of the girls we talked with said they were unhappy with their bodies. And most admitted to us that they really don't know what the best way is for teenagers to lose weight. The best way is definitely *not* a diet designed for adults, whose nutritional needs are vastly different from yours. You need a special diet designed for teenagers only.

Now some of you may actually need to drop a few pounds, while others may just need a better body image reality check. Either way, chances are you could be eating a lot smarter nutritionally, which means you need to know a few things about what's happening to you.

RIGHT NOW, YOU ARE IN THE BIGGEST, MOST CRITICAL GROWTH SPURT OF YOUR LIFE.

You've probably been through puberty or are in the last phases of it. During puberty (when the body "grows up" and is capable of giving birth) the bones in your legs and arms grow long, hips widen, breasts develop, you get curvier, hair grows in new places, your waist becomes fuller, and you gain some weight.

It may feel weird to be filling out, like maybe you're getting fat, but remember it's normal. Without this change, you wouldn't have periods or ever be able to have babies!

Your body is also releasing hormones like estrogen, FHS (follicle-stimulating hormone), and LH (luteinizing hormone). They can affect your moods as well as your energy levels. It's really an incredible process when you think about it. But because of all these growth and hormone changes, it can be a tough time to diet.

BEFORE PUBERTY, GIRLS HAVE ABOUT 19 PERCENT BODY FAT. AFTER PUBERTY, GIRLS HAVE ABOUT 22 PERCENT.

Believe it or not, **YOU ACTUALLY REQUIRE *MORE* CALORIES THAN NORMAL RIGHT NOW, ONES WITH "NUTRIENT DENSITY."** (These are foods that give you more nutritional bang for your buck.) Yeah, you heard that right! Technically, your body needs *more* fuel right now, so the quality of what you put in your mouth is critical. You are laying the groundwork for how healthy you'll be for the rest of your life. Your bones—your body's foundation—grow in length and density mostly during your teens. Strong bones now will mean strong bones when you're a cute little old lady!

So if your body needs more fuel right now, why are we writing a diet book? Because there's a difference between the weight and curviness you're *supposed* to gain and what lots of teenagers are *really* gaining.

Here are some pretty amazing statistics. Recent research shows that 31 percent of American teenage girls are somewhat overweight and an additional 15 percent are obese. Yet another recent study shows that overweight teenagers have an 80 percent chance of becoming overweight adults!

If you're really overweight, then this diet will help you lose weight without shortchanging your body's nutritional needs. We want you to diet responsibly so you don't hurt yourself nutritionally. Even if you don't need to diet, you'll learn a lot about nutrition from this book. Either way, you're smart to want to develop great eating habits now that will benefit you for the rest of your life.

Truth be told, some of you may be packing on pounds because you simply eat too much, eat the wrong stuff, or don't exercise. Some people might blame you, but we think there's plenty of blame to go around!

It's never been tougher to eat right. Marketers are bombarding you with ads for super-sizing and junk foods. Magazines and TV are showcasing impossibly thin people. And either you're too busy to eat well on a consistent basis, or you don't have a lot going on—leaving you bored, lonely, or depressed. The consequences? You're not making good food choices. Add Mother Nature, who's forcing your body to gain weight, and you're in a pickle!

The goal here is *not* to derail Mother Nature's plan and put yourself in a health-risk situation. Not eating enough of the right foods will hurt you. But overeating and eating the wrong foods will also cause health risks— serious ones that will only get worse as you grow older.

FACT: BEING OVERWEIGHT IS DANGEROUS

Here's why. Your bones, heart, and lungs need to work harder when you're carrying extra pounds of body fat. Sure, you may feel basically okay, but you are straining your body systems. Plus you're a sitting duck for health problems like:

 Diabetes

 Heart disease

 Gallbladder disease

 High blood pressure

 Respiratory problems

 Osteoporosis

Not good. Here's a cold, hard fact. If you're overweight, it's because of one or more of these reasons:

 You eat too much.

 You don't work out.

You have a medical condition, like an endocrine disorder or hormone imbalance. (These medical conditions are rare, but serious. We strongly suggest that you check with a doctor before you start any diet. Your doctor may need to test your hormone levels.)

Once you've got a doctor's okay, there is only one way to lose weight safely. No magic pills, no special supplements, no fad diets. It's very simple. Your body weight is controlled by two things: how many calories you eat and how many you burn.

IN ORDER TO LOSE WEIGHT, YOU HAVE TO BURN OFF MORE CALORIES THAN YOU EAT.

If you're serious about losing weight and eating right, you'll need to do a few things. Let's start with this: forget everything you've heard about what you should and shouldn't eat and what's good for you and what's not. Chances are, all that stuff applies to adults—not necessarily to you. As a teenager, you have special needs right now. (You'll find out exactly what they are in the next chapter.)

So empty your mind of all the stuff you've heard before about eating and dieting. We're going to start with some new basics.

1. **Carbs (carbohydrates) aren't bad. You need them to make your brain work!**

2. **How *much* you eat is as important as *what* you eat.**

3. **Don't deprive yourself, and never exclude a food group.**

4. **Always eat breakfast.**

5. **Avoid soda! Diet soda, too! They can cause cellulite and bloating—ugh!**

6. **Avoid artificial sweeteners.**

7. **Avoid hydrogenated oils.**

8. **Avoid processed foods (anything with lots of white flour and sugars and oils, like cookies, crackers, and baked goods).**

9. Avoid high fructose corn syrup (sweetener found in juices and other drinks).

10. Have your meals get SMALLER as the day goes on.

There will be lots more advice and secrets to come, but these are the big ones to get started with as you retrain your brain and learn the truth about what your body really needs when it comes to eating right. Remember, it's not easy to lose weight. If it were, everyone would be in great shape!

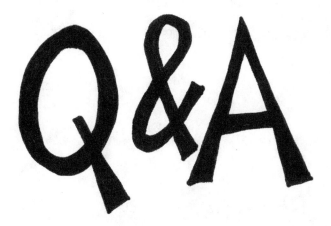

I'M EMBARRASSED TO ASK THIS, BUT WHAT EXACTLY IS A CARB OR CARBOHYDRATE?

No worries, we don't expect you to know this stuff! Here's the technical definition (for science class!): carbohydrates are an organic compound made up of carbon, hydrogen, and oxygen. Now for the easy definition: carbohydrates are foods like grains, legumes (beans and lentils), starchy vegetables, and fruits.

SHOULD I EAT LOW-CALORIE OR LOW-CARB FOODS?

If you have to choose, opt for a low-calorie diet. Diets that limit your carbo-hydrate intake (foods like breads and pastas) will help you lose *water* weight. What you really want to lose is body fat.

On a low-calorie diet, watch out that you don't go too low and cut out important nutrients. We recommend that you stick to our guidelines when it comes to the number of calories you want to eat to lose weight. (You'll find out in chapter 4!)

ARE DIETS LIKE ATKINS OR SOUTH BEACH OKAY FOR ME? AND HOW DO THOSE DIETS WORK ANYWAY?

What we don't like about these low-carb diets, in general, is that they're asking you to avoid food groups containing vital nutrients that you need right now. For example, you don't see lots of calcium-rich foods in the Atkins Diet. And you see very little fruit (which is linked to the prevention of cancer and heart disease) in the South Beach Diet.

In general, these diets rob your body of carbohydrates, so your body has to get energy from fat and protein. This puts your body in an altered state called *ketosis*. You shed stored body water, which looks impressive on the scale, but can actually be harmful to your health. In the short run, ketosis can cause acid breath, dehydration, fuzzy thinking, fatigue, and constipation. In the long run, it can cause serious damage— like muscle and bone loss, kidney and liver problems, and diabetes.

Also keep in mind that on "fad" diets like these (the kinds that promise quick weight loss), you'll easily regain any water weight that you lose once you start eating normally again. A good diet, like this diet for teens, will target the fat stores in your body to help you lose weight permanently.

WHAT ABOUT THE RAW DIET? I HAVE FRIENDS ON THAT.

The premise of this one is that by cooking foods they lose their nutrient value, so you should eat raw foods. In fact, some foods like carrots and tomatoes are easier for the body to absorb if they are cooked. We don't recommend the Raw Diet for teenagers because it doesn't focus enough on your calcium and iron intake, which is so important at your age.

SHOULD I USE DIET AIDS?

No. Here's why: First, the ones that act as laxatives can be addictive to the point where you become desensitized and don't know when you need to go to the bathroom! Second, fat burners and diet pills are basically speeding up your metabolism with ingredients like caffeine and herbs. These herbs can be dangerous, especially if you mix them with the wrong food or medicine! For example, ginseng can cause low blood sugar and toxicity syndrome, as well as hypertension and nervousness. Saint John's wort can counteract the effectiveness of birth control pills and cancer-fighting drugs. The active ingredient called *bitter orange* found in some ephedra weight-loss alternatives has been shown to increase the risk of high blood pressure, heart attacks, and strokes.

IS IT OKAY TO EAT VEGETARIAN? CAN I DO THAT ON THIS DIET?

Yes! And yes! It's fine to be a vegetarian as long as you get the right combo of protein, grains, and legumes, plus adequate vitamins and minerals. (See the next chapter!)

Remember, your body is your friend. Celebrate what it can do, how it allows you to lead an active and healthy life. Don't get sucked in by magazine and media standards of "thin" people and how you *should* look. These are screwy social standards that make virtually everyone feel inadequate. You're not. You deserve to feel good about yourself, how you look, and the way you eat.

TAKE CARE OF YOUR BODY. AFTER ALL, IT'S THE ONLY PLACE YOU'LL HAVE TO LIVE!

—JIM ROHN, MOTIVATIONAL SPEAKER

THE *TWO* DAILY SIX FOR CHICKS

Wanna know what the daily six are? They're the nutrients your body needs every day. Still got that pen or pencil handy? We'd like you to jot down what you think those six vital nutrients are. (Don't feel bad if you don't get this—most people don't!)

1. _____

2. _____

3. _____

4. _____

5. _____

6. _____

How did you do? Turn the page to find out . . .

THE DAILY SIX NUTRIENTS ARE:

1. **Carbohydrates**

2. **Proteins**

3. **Fats**

4. **Minerals**

5. **Vitamins**

6. **Water**

Basically speaking, your body needs all of these nutrients in order to keep functioning correctly. Literally. Nutrients supply the energy that keeps your heart beating and the ingredients that keep your brain active, plus they keep your muscles working. They also provide the structure to build bones, muscles, and tendons. And miraculously, they regulate entire body processes, like maintaining body temperature and carrying oxygen through your blood. Impressive, right?

Now that you know how *important* all of these nutrients are, let's talk about how each of them makes your body operate.

1. CARBOHYDRATES

Carbs come in two forms, complex and simple.

☆ **COMPLEX CARBS** are better for you because your body digests them more slowly and they don't spike your blood sugar. These carbs would rather be used as energy than stored as fat. (Good sources: whole grains, brown rice, yams, lentils, beans, and most vegetables and fruits.)

☆ **SIMPLE CARBS** such as table sugar or refined flour are the ones you want to limit because they will spike your blood sugar—meaning, they'll cause a rush of insulin to be dumped into your bloodstream. That will make you crave more sugary foods, sending you in a vicious cycle that will sap your energy and make you want to eat more food to bring your energy back up. And that can result in weight gain!

NOW, COMMIT THIS TO MEMORY: THE RIGHT CARBS ARE GOOD FOR YOU!

Carbs are the exclusive fuel for the brain. Plus they fuel the nervous system and power fat metabolism! Without carbs, you can have symptoms like this:

 Foggy thinking

 Fatigue

 Moodiness

 Constipation

 Bad breath

Yuck. So if you've been brainwashed into thinking "carbs are bad," banish that thought. Your body and your brain need those carbohydrates!

2. PROTEINS

You probably already have a good idea of what proteins are—meats, poultry, eggs, fish, and dairy. But do you know what they do for you and why they're vital to your health? Proteins make up your organs, tissues, blood, hormonal and immune systems, skin, and other body parts. They also contain the building blocks called amino acids, which help your cells produce energy and hormones.

3. FATS

Fats come in many forms—monounsaturated, polyunsaturated, saturated . . . oh man, this can get confusing! And what are trans fats anyway? We shall explain!

But let's keep it simple. First of all, you need some fat in your diet. True story. So get the "fat is bad" out of your diet vocabulary. You need some fat to keep your body parts well oiled and to pad your vital organs to keep them protected. For example, do you ever envy other girls' shiny hair and healthy looking skin? Guess what, they're getting the right kinds of fat in their diet—omega–3's help keep skin and hair healthy and beautiful. (More on omega–3-rich foods at the end of this chapter.)

But let's get back to the basics of what *kinds* of fat you should and shouldn't be putting inside that beautiful body machine of yours.

⭑ MONOUNSATURATED FATS You want to gravitate toward these because they lower the bad cholesterol and raise the good cholesterol, which help prevent heart disease and certain cancers. (Good sources: olive oils, nut oils, canola oil, olives, and avocados.)

⭑ POLYUNSATURATED FATS These are good for you because they're heart protectors and may reduce the risk of certain cancers, too. (Good sources: vegetable oils like corn, sunflower, and fish oils.)

☆ SATURATED FATS You'll find these in animal products, whole milk, and tropical oils. You know how fat on steak gets solid at room temperature? That's saturated fat. If you eat a lot of this kind of fat, you risk raising your blood cholesterol levels which could block your arteries and cause heart attacks—not so healthy. Try to eat lean meats and low- or nonfat dairy products.

☆ TRANS FATS They're not good for you and are kind of like saturated fats. Trans fats are a type of fatty acid that forms during a process called hydrogenation (which manufacturers use to make their foods last longer on the shelf). Good for shelf life, not for your life!

4. MINERALS

Minerals are also found in foods but only in very small amounts in most diets. That's why taking a daily mineral supplement is a great idea. Some minerals that are especially important for you during this growing period are iron, calcium, and magnesium.

IRON IS VITAL FOR MAKING YOUR RED BLOOD CELLS. YOU LOSE A LOT OF IRON DURING YOUR PERIOD.

You can get this mineral in iron-rich foods like wheat germ or dark green vegetables. The daily suggested amount is 18 mgs.

CALCIUM IS CRITICAL FOR YOUR DEVELOPMENT RIGHT NOW, ESPECIALLY FOR YOUR BONES AND TEETH!

Did you know your bones are still forming in your teens? By the time you're seventeen, almost all (90 percent) of your bones have developed. So be good to them now, and they'll be good to you when you get older! Plus—*newsflash!*—the latest research shows that calcium might *prevent fat storage* by intercepting it with a special mechanism in the body.

CALCIUM = MAGIC DIET BULLET!

Here's what we want you to do. Make sure you get three servings *per day* of non- or low-fat dairy foods. You need 1200 mgs of calcium per day. So if you follow this diet and have a cup of low-fat milk or low-fat yogurt and a piece of low-fat cheese, you'll have most of what you need. Then take a supplement that contains 600 mgs of calcium citrate (make sure it's calcium *citrate*—it's easier for your body to absorb) with 300 mgs of

21

magnesium and some vitamin D. These help your body absorb calcium. *Hint:* Take the calcium/magnesium at night—it can help make you sleepy.

5. VITAMINS

Vitamins work at a cellular level in your body to help metabolize the nutrients from food. In other words, they help release the nutrients more efficiently so that they're more easily absorbed into your bloodstream. Sadly, most teenagers (and many adults!) aren't getting the right amounts of vitamins and minerals in their diets—meaning they aren't as healthy as they could be. Essential vitamins for you are A, B (several kinds), C, D, and E. With the exception of vitamin D and a little bit of vitamin K, your body does not make vitamins.

VITAMIN A is important for healthy skin, hair, bones, and eyes. You will find vitamin A in milk, eggs, liver, carrots, and other orange fruits and vegetables.

VITAMIN B'S help keep your heart, muscles, and nervous system working correctly. There are several B vitamins: B_1 (thiamin), B_2 (riboflavin), B_3 (niacin), B_5, B_6, B_9 (folic acid), and B_{12}. B_5 is often used to treat PMS (premenstrual syndrome); B_9 is critical for pregnant women; and B_{12} helps with red blood cell formation. B vitamins are found in lots of foods, including

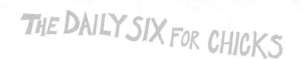

whole grains, peanut butter, fish, peas, soy foods, potatoes, bananas, eggs, wheat germ, citrus fruit, chicken, and spinach.

VITAMIN C is sometimes called ascorbic acid. It helps heal wounds, and is important for healthy teeth, gums, and brain function. The best sources of vitamin C are kiwis, green peppers, tomatoes, broccoli, spinach, oranges, and grapefruit.

VITAMIN D helps the body absorb calcium and is critical for your developing bones. Good sources? The sun, (that's why vitamin D is sometimes called the sunshine vitamin), egg yolks, and fish oils.

VITAMIN E keeps your nervous and immune systems running smoothly. It also helps make red blood cells healthy. Good sources are nuts, leafy green vegetables, wheat germ, and avocados.

VITAMIN K is important for blood clotting, which helps your body heal cuts and wounds. Vitamin K can be found in liver, eggs, and green leafy vegetables.

The best way to get your daily dose of vitamins and minerals is to eat a balanced diet. If you aren't eating well, doctors recommend an ordinary daily multivitamin supplement. This diet will provide for all your daily needs, but since your calorie intake will be lower, it'll be a good idea to include a multivitamin.

NOTE OF CAUTION

Taking large doses of vitamins is not a good idea. Water-soluble vitamins like C can leave your body through urine or sweat. But fat-soluble vitamins like A, D, E, and K can build up in your body and cause serious problems. For example, if you're taking oral acne medications, you're already getting lots of vitamin A. If you take extra A, you can overdose on it and suffer side effects like blurred vision, hair loss, or liver damage. Don't take extra vitamin A if you're on oral acne medications!

6. WATER

Did you know that most of your body—approximately 65 percent of it—is composed of water? Your brain is actually three-quarters water! So H_2O is the most important power nutrient. Without enough water, nutrients like carbs, proteins, and fats can't get into your body's cells.

Water is critical for weight loss because it helps flush out toxins and keeps you hydrated, giving you beautiful skin and a healthy body!

You should drink approximately 2 quarts (64 ounces) of water a day. That's the same as 8 medium-size glasses every day. (Did you know that sometimes *your body can confuse hunger with thirst*? If you're hungry, try drinking something first.)

Also, we like some of the bottled waters you can buy in stores, like the brand called Fruit Waters by Glacéau. (Don't confuse them with the same company's "Vitamin Waters," which have sugar in them.) Calistoga flavored waters and plain decaf iced teas are good, too. Another way to make water more interesting is to do what they do at exclusive health spas. Put regular water in a pitcher with cut up cucumbers, lemons, and oranges. Pour and enjoy. Very tasty!

There are two more "wonder workers" that help round out your diet: phytochemicals and fiber.

PHYTOCHEMICALS (ALSO KNOWN AS ANTIOXIDANTS)

They're not vitamins or minerals but compounds found in fruits and vegetables. They can help prevent heart disease and cancer by neutralizing free radicals that damage cell walls. Since some cancers can take 20 to 30 years to become full blown, you're never too young to take super good care of yourself!

You'll find these incredible disease-fighting compounds in vitamins C, E, and beta-carotene (vitamin A). You'll also find them in foods like broccoli; cabbage; Brussels sprouts; onions; garlic; yellow, orange, or red fruits and vegetables; dark greens; citrus fruits; soybeans; and whole grain cereals. Eat your vegetables, darlin'!

FIBER

There are two kinds of fiber, soluble and insoluble. **Soluble fiber** (like celery, beets, lentils, and whole grains) goes through your digestive system intact, cleaning it out like a Brillo pad. **Insoluble fiber** (like the roughage from vegetables) stimulates your digestive system and gives you a pretty immediate feeling of being full—because it absorbs water.

Fiber also slows down the release of glucose (blood sugar) into the bloodstream, which leaves you satisfied longer after eating it. Studies have shown that people who eat fiber at breakfast (like wheat bran) eat less food throughout the day.

Here's a fascinating fact: good fiber intake lowers the risk of breast cancer! A recent study about teens and fiber shows that good fiber intake reduces the amount of circulating estrogen, which is generally high during puberty. *Lower* levels of circulating estrogen mean a *lower* risk of cancer later in life.

Giving your body the right nutrition in the right amounts can make a huge difference in your life and, frankly, in your moods. Our hope is for you to establish a healthy relationship with food. Once you really understand how important nutrition is and how it can nurture you, you will see food as a friend, not an enemy. Food should be an enjoyable and healthy part of your life.

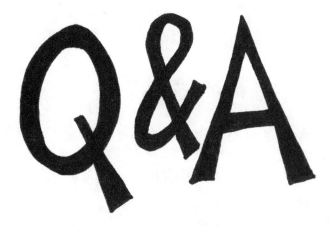

Q&A

IS IT BETTER TO EAT THREE BIG MEALS OR LOTS OF SMALLER ONES DURING THE DAY?

For this diet, it's better to eat three average-size meals and snack throughout the day to keep your body running smoothly and to make sure you're getting the right nutrients.

SHOULD I TAKE VITAMINS?

Sure! You get most of what you need by eating right. But when you diet and reduce calories, you may be limiting certain vitamins. Ask a pharmacist to recommend a good daily multivitamin for you.

WHAT PERCENT FAT MILK SHOULD I DRINK?

Nonfat or 1 percent.

WHAT IF I CAN'T DRINK MILK?

You must get your calcium in different forms:

* **Drink lactose-free milk (without the milk sugar that your body can't digest).**

* **Take a lactose digestive aid tablet like Lacteez before eating dairy products.**

* **Eat calcium-rich foods like broccoli, sardines, or fortified orange juice.**

* **Take a calcium/magnesium supplement.**

DOES LOW-FAT MEAN LOW-CALORIE?

Nope! And don't let those manufacturers fool you. Many low-fat and nonfat foods replace the fat with carbohydrates, which means the number of calories aren't actually reduced! Tricky, eh? So check the label for the calorie amount and compare it with that of a regular nondiet product.

HOW MUCH FIBER SHOULD I GET A DAY?

About 25 grams per day. Here's how much you will find in a single serving of any of the following foods (just to name a few).

Baked beans ....8.9 grams

Lentils ....7.3 grams

Wild rice ....4 grams

Wheat pasta............4 grams

Asian pear ....4 grams

Orange.....................4 grams

Instant cocoa ....3 grams

WHAT SHOULD MY DAILY LIMIT OF SALT (SODIUM) BE?

About 2000 mgs. Watch out for products with super-high concentrations of salt—like some soups, frozen foods, and fast foods. Too much salt is associated with the risk of high blood pressure. If you have a medical condition called *hypertension*, you should be eating even less sodium. Talk to your doctor about this.

WHAT ARE THE OMEGA OILS I KEEP HEARING ABOUT?

There are omega–3's and omega–6's. The technical name for omega–3 is alpha linolenic acid. You'll find the omega–3's in coldwater fish like salmon, tuna, and cod, and in flaxseed, walnuts, and wheat germ. Studies show that if you get omega–3's early in life (that is, right now!), they can actually help *prevent* the development of excessive numbers of fat cells. Yeah, you heard that right—eat nutritiously now and you can keep fat away later in life!

The technical name for omega–6's is lineloic acid. You'll find these in sunflower, safflower, and corn oils, as well as in the supplement called evening primrose oil (which can reduce symptoms of PMS, or premenstrual syndrome).

In general, these omega oils increase your metabolism and help *burn* fat instead of *storing* it!

HOW DO YOU FEEL ABOUT FAT SUBSTITUTES, LIKE THIS OLESTRA STUFF I'VE SEEN IN POTATO CHIPS?

It would be great if Olestra or other substitutes were tasty and good for dieting, but so far there's been lots of controversy surrounding them. The concern is that these fats might hinder the body from absorbing nutrients

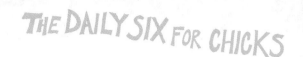

and vitamins. Plus many people are reporting digestive problems, like cramps and diarrhea. For this diet, we say stay away from products with fat substitutes in them.

WHAT ARE ANTIOXIDANTS?

These are groups of compounds found in foods like fruits and vegetables and certain teas. They help neutralize free radicals (atoms) that get into your system and damage cells.

In this diet, our favorite source of antioxidants is called Pom Tea! The secret recipe is coming up in chapter 5!

IS IT OKAY TO FAST? IT SOUNDS KIND OF COOL TO "CLEANSE" YOUR SYSTEM.

We don't recommend it for you, especially because long-term fasts can be dangerous because you're not getting vital nutrients. If you're interested in fasting because you've heard that they "detox" or cleanse your system try other ways to do that—by eating clear broths or soups and liquids containing fruits and vegetables for no more than two consecutive days. No scientific studies have proven that fasts are good for you.

Okay, now that you know the essentials about nutrition, let's find out in the next chapter whether you need to lose weight or just some pre-conceived notions about how you *think* you should look!

FOOD FOR THOUGHT: DON'T LET YOUR STOMACH BE A WAIST BASKET.

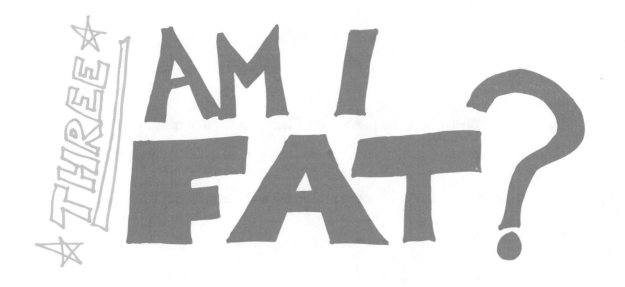

THREE ☆ AM I FAT?

I REMEMBER THE EXACT MOMENT WHEN I BECAME AWARE OF MY BODY AND WEIGHT. I WAS ABOUT ELEVEN, MY DANCE TEACHER WAS LOOKING RIGHT AT ME AND SAID, "SUCK IN YOUR STOMACH."
—TEENAGER

So it begins—your relationship with your body weight. And as most women do at some time in their lives, you ask: Wait . . . *am I fat*??? The answer depends on a lot of different factors. In just a moment, we'll help

33

you find out (using a special formula) if you're really overweight and if your body image matches reality.

But before you make a decision to lose weight, make a pact with yourself. Your lifestyle and eating habits are going to change. Keep in mind:

1. **You'll need to be patient. (This isn't just another quick-fix weight-loss diet, although you'll see great results immediately.)**

2. **You'll need to be more physically and mentally active.**

3. **You'll need to plan your meals and snacks.**

While you're getting ready to go through all these changes, there is one diet trick that really works and you can start it right now! It's a food diary. We've got one for you at the end of the book [page 223]. Keep track of what you're eating, how much water you're drinking and, most importantly, how you're feeling. It's been proven that people who keep a food diary are more successful at losing weight than those who don't. Plus, the diary helps you really see your eating habits and diet progress.

Okay, now for the answer to that burning question: are you fat? One of the best ways to find out what kind of shape you're in is to use a scientific formula called BMI (Body Mass Index). This is the most recognized method used to determine the amount of body fat you have.

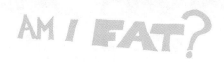

Here's how to find out your own personal BMI number (hey, that math you learned is finally coming in handy!).

1. Divide your weight in pounds by your height in inches.

2. Divide the answer from step 1 by your height in inches.

3. Multiply your answer from step 2 by 703. That's your BMI!

REMEMBER YOUR BMI NUMBER! YOU'LL NEED IT LATER!

NOTE: REMEMBER, LOTS OF DIFFERENT FACTORS MAY AFFECT YOUR BMI. FOR EXAMPLE, IT'S NORMAL FOR GIRLS (AND GUYS!) TO GAIN WEIGHT RAPIDLY DURING THEIR TEENAGE YEARS, AND ALMOST EVERYONE'S BMI NUMBER JUMPS UP DURING PUBERTY. ALSO, IF YOU'RE A BIG PERSON WITH LARGE BONES, YOUR BMI COULD BE HIGH EVEN THOUGH YOU DON'T HAVE EXCESS FAT. LIKEWISE, IF YOU'RE LITTLE AND SMALL BONED, YOU COULD HAVE A REGULAR BMI NUMBER YET STILL HAVE TOO MUCH BODY FAT. THAT'S WHY IT'S GREAT TO CHECK WITH A DOCTOR. HE OR SHE CAN HELP YOU FIGURE OUT IF YOU'RE REALLY OVER-WEIGHT AND NEED TO LOSE SOME POUNDS, AND WHETHER ANY RECENT WEIGHT GAIN IS NORMAL OR NEEDS MORE ATTENTION.

Now that you have your personal BMI number, find it in the row next to your age group to find out if you're in the fit, slightly overweight, overweight, or obese category. (Just so you know, we've taken the numbers and adjusted them for your age groups based on scientific studies and growth charts designed specifically for teenage girls.)

AGE	FIT	SLIGHTLY OVERWEIGHT	OVERWEIGHT	OBESE
13–14	19–20	21–23	24–25	26+
15–16	20–21	22–24	25–28	29+
17–19	21–22	23–25	26–29	30+

No panicking allowed if you're in the last three columns. It just means you can choose to do something about your weight if you want to be more fit. You need a plan, a sane one. Quick knee-jerk reactions like "Oh my God I have to lose weight now!" are common but unproductive. Follow that up with: "I will lose weight the *right* way." And think: "I may not have a weight problem, but an *eating* problem." This diet will help you eliminate those problems.

We don't expect you to know how to lose weight and diet safely—it's not like anyone teaches you that in class. Nor do we expect you to

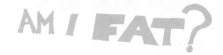

learn everything you need to know and get fit overnight. But it will happen if you're dedicated and serious about treating yourself right.

By now you've probably asked yourself: **how much should I weigh?** The answer to that is: you should be at a weight that's healthy for you. That doesn't necessarily mean it's the weight at which you are your slimmest. It's the weight that works for you—the one at which you will actually look and feel your best. Don't confuse the two! We want you to be healthy!

Your healthy weight is determined by lots of things and has to take into account variables like body fat, muscle, bone structure, and genetics that are specific to your body type. It can be normal for the two people who are the same height to have very different healthy weights. To find out how much you should weigh, it's best to go to a doctor who has kept track of your height and weight since you were little.

Just remember, weight is only one measurement of health; sometimes a skinny person isn't as healthy as someone who's heavier. Health has to do with good nutrition, fitness, and feeling good in your body.

Now your next question is probably: **if I really need to lose weight, how should I do it?** If you do decide you want to diet, there's only one safe and sane way to go about it. You need a plan that's right for you—a plan that focuses on a variety of foods, portion control, and exercise. Steer clear of diet aids or fad weight-loss tricks. Do it the right, healthy, nutritional way.

BOTTOM LINE:
FEWER CALORIES + MORE EXERCISE = WEIGHT LOSS

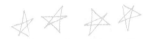

That means you need to know how many calories you should be eating a day in order to lose weight. Generally speaking, you need to eat about 500 calories less a day than you're currently eating in order to lose a pound a week. Coming up in the next chapter is the actual diet, where you'll find out exactly the number of calories recommended for you based on your BMI number. (You remember yours, right?)

But before you decide to diet, you need to be really honest with yourself. Are you really overweight or are you super critical of yourself? Your BMI number and fitness chart on page 36 can help give you a reality check. So can a doctor, a dietician, or a nutritionist.

We don't want you to diet if you're doing it just for looks. Most young women worry more about how they *look* when they're overweight than how *healthy* they are. **We want you to care more about how healthy and fit you are.** If you are significantly overweight, though, you have an increased risk of developing health problems like diabetes and high blood pressure. Overweight teens are more likely to become overweight adults. If you are in the fit column, you can still use this book to

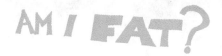

learn how to eat right and get the nutrition your body needs. Keep in mind that the average teenager needs anywhere from 2000 to 2600 calories a day, depending on her body's needs.

The last thing we want is for you to have to deal with dieting and food and health issues for the rest of your life. If you can learn about nutrition and create good eating habits now, you could be saving yourself a lifetime of hassles. It would be great if you could avoid the pain that millions of women before you have had to go through!

Now here's something we want you to try: never again ask yourself the question "Am I fat?" Seriously. We have a better question for you. Instead of asking "Am I fat?" we want you to ask "Am I *fit*?"—as in, "Am I healthy and in shape?" That's what you should be striving for.

Some people have naturally larger builds and aren't meant to be skinny minnies. If you are one of them, accept it and move on to being as healthy and beautiful as you can be. The skinny, pretty women in this world aren't always the most attractive. The supremely confident and healthy woman who knows how to carry herself and take care of herself is *really* the most attractive.

If you do decide you need to lose weight, the next chapter is your safe, sane way to do it! Your life is about to change in a big way—in the way you eat, the way you think of yourself, the way you take care of yourself, and the way you talk to yourself. Here are some new strategies to start you off!

INSTEAD OF SAYING:	SAY:
I'M FAT.	I'M GOING TO BE FIT.
EVERYONE IS SKINNIER THAN ME.	I WILL HONOR THE BODY I HAVE.
NO ONE THINKS I'M HOT.	I WILL ACCEPT AND LOVE MYSELF AS I AM. I THINK I'M HOT!
I CAN'T DO IT. I'M A FAILURE.	I WANT SOMETHING BETTER FOR MYSELF. ALL I ASK OF MYSELF IS TO TRY. REALLY TRY—NOT JUST PRETEND AND THEN WHINE.
WOW, THAT AD SAYS I CAN LOSE LOTS OF WEIGHT ON THEIR DIET. I WANT THAT.	OH REALLY? WHAT KIND OF WEIGHT WOULD I BE LOSING, WATER WEIGHT OR REAL WEIGHT? THERE ARE NO QUICK FIXES.

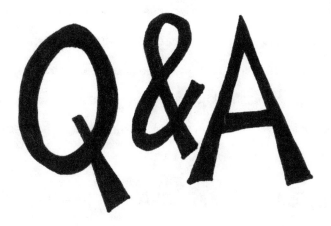

Q&A

JUST WHAT IS A CALORIE ANYWAY?

Calories measure energy in food and in your body. You can impress your science teacher by telling her/him that one calorie is the amount of energy necessary to raise the temperature of water by 1 degree centigrade. Now aren't you the smart one! Going for extra credit? Then you can add that scientists measure calories using an instrument called a bomb calorimeter. They put food inside the machine, surround it with water, and then burn it! The heat released raises the temperature of the water in the box, so if it goes up 10 centigrade degrees, then the food is 10 calories.

ARE THERE SUCH THINGS AS EMPTY CALORIES?

Yes. They're calories that have no nutritional value, like the calories in cola drinks. They're not good for you because these drinks are filled with sugar and caffeine. The opposite of empty calories are nutrient-dense calories. For example, a piece of fruit that gives you fiber, vitamins, and minerals has the kind of calories you should be allowing into your body! Empty calories aren't healthful fuel; all they do is add up to more weight and less energy.

I WANT TO LOSE 10 POUNDS. WHAT'S THE BEST WAY TO DO THAT?

Go on this diet or consult a doctor, dietician, or nutritionist who can put you on a healthy eating plan that's right for you. And make sure you exercise!

HOW ABOUT IF I JUST DON'T EAT, OR CUT WAY BACK ON CALORIES? I KNOW I'LL LOSE WEIGHT.

WATCH OUT! This strategy could backfire on you. When you really go low on the calories, you body's metabolic rate (i.e. how well your body burns fuel/calories) adapts quickly to conserve the fewer calories you are taking in. So don't ever cut your intake drastically. Chances are, you won't lose weight any faster that way than if you're on a good diet.

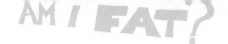

MY MOM BOUGHT SOMETHING CALLED HOLLYWOOD DRINK THAT HELPS HER LOSE WEIGHT IN 48 HOURS. SHOULD I ALSO TRY IT?

No! You would only be losing water weight. Not fat.

I HATE EATING BREAKFAST BECAUSE I'M ALWAYS IN A RUSH. CAN I JUST SKIP IT?

No, we highly recommend you eat breakfast. Think of it like this: you are *break*ing a *fast* in the morning—that is, you haven't fed your body since the night before. Your body needs to get jump started in the morning so that it can start burning calories. People who don't eat breakfast tend to overeat later in the day because they get ravenous. Eat breakfast and your body will burn calories more efficiently throughout the rest of the day!

HOW OFTEN SHOULD I WEIGH MYSELF?

Weigh yourself at the beginning of your diet, preferably in the morning and then no more often than every 7 to 10 days. Scales are a useful tool, but they can give you misleading information if you're constantly weighing yourself. Daily weight checks will just create a nasty cycle. For example, if you eat a lot of salt one day and retain water weight the next, you might think you've gained weight when you really haven't.

SHOULD I MEASURE MYSELF?

Yes! This is a far better way to see your progress, particularly for girls. You'll see your weight loss reflected more in inches than in pounds on this diet, especially if you exercise. Check out the measuring chart that we've provided for you at the end of this book [see page 230], and try it for the next few weeks!

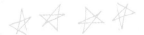

I AM BEAUTIFUL, NO MATTER WHAT THEY SAY . . . WORDS WON'T BRING ME DOWN.

—FROM THE SONG "BEAUTIFUL" PERFORMED BY CHRISTINA AGUILERA

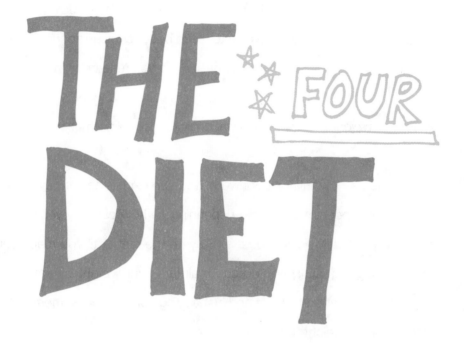

THE DIET

Okay, here it is. The diet for teenagers only. The magic key to this diet is simple: **knowing how big a serving size really is and understanding nutrition.**

This diet is not about starving or depriving yourself. That doesn't work in the long run. In fact, a recent article in the journal *Pediatrics* confirms that teenagers on restrictive diets end up gaining more weight than on nonrestrictive diets or no diet at all. Why? Because strict diets are hard to stay on—people get hungry and tend to overeat once they're off the diet.

On this diet you'll get to eat your favorite foods, including dessert, pizza, and chips. But you'll be able to make better choices about *what* you eat, and *how much* of it, thanks to everything you're learning about nutrition and serving sizes. Once you understand this diet and follow it carefully, you'll *lose weight* and *gain intelligence* about food—information that you'll use forever.

Here's how this diet will work. You can expect an average weight loss of 1 to 5 pounds per week, depending on how carefully you follow it and how physically active you are. Stay on the diet until you reach your healthy weight goal. Then you can maintain your weight by eating the same way you eat on this diet and just adding some calories (more details on maintaining weight to come).

Here's what's going to happen in this chapter.

 We'll help you find out how many calories (1400, 1600, or 2000) you'll need to eat per day in order to lose weight.

 You'll see what a balanced diet looks like and how the diet works.

 We'll "show & tell" you how big one serving of food really is.

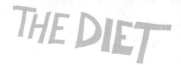

⭐ And finally, we'll give you the 7-day meal plans and vegetarian alternatives for this diet.

FIND YOUR CALORIE CATEGORY

To figure out *your* calorie category (or how many calories a day you'll need to eat in order to lose weight) you will need to plug your BMI number from chapter 3 into this next chart.

In case you forgot your BMI number, here's the formula again.

1. **Divide your weight by your height in inches.**

2. **Divide the answer from step 1 by your height in inches.**

3. **Multiply your answer from step 2 by 703. That's your BMI!**

Now, find your age group in the first column of the chart on the next page. Then scan the second column to find your BMI number. Finally, find your calorie category in the third column, and—bingo—that's the number of calories you're going to be eating per day in order to lose weight.

AGE	BMI	CALORIE CATEGORY
13-14	21-23	1400
	24-25	1600
	26+	2000
15-16	22-24	1400
	25-28	1600
	29+	2000
17-19	23-25	1400
	26-29	1600
	30+	2000

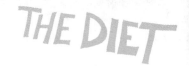

WHAT A BALANCED DIET LOOKS LIKE

Your diet needs to be nutritionally rich and well-balanced for your body, especially during these critical years while you're growing and setting the stage for lifelong eating habits. The following daily nutrition percentages are built into our diet plans:

30% PROTEINS

30% OF YOUR DAILY NUTRITION COMES FROM THE PROTEIN GROUP, WHICH INCLUDES DAIRY.

50% CARBS

50% OF YOUR DAILY NUTRITION COMES FROM CARBOHYDRATES LIKE GRAINS, LEGUMES, STARCHY AND GREEN VEGGIES, AND FRUITS.

20% FATS

20% OF YOUR DAILY NUTRITION COMES FROM FATS, INCLUDING SNACKS AND CONDIMENTS.

HERE'S HOW THAT BALANCED DIET BREAKS DOWN INTO DIFFERENT FOOD GROUPS.

 1. THE G GROUP: Grains, legumes, and starchy vegetables (grains are foods like breads and cereals; legumes are foods like beans and lentils; starchy veggies are foods like potatoes and yams; green veggies like broccoli and cucumbers will be "free"—meaning they won't count in your calorie total.)

 2. THE F GROUP: Fruits (fresh whole fruit and fruit juices)

 3. THE D GROUP: Dairy (low- or nonfat milk, yogurt, cheese)

 4. THE P GROUP: Proteins (meat, fish, chicken, tuna, egg whites)

 5. THE S GROUP: Snacks (crackers, popcorn, peanut butter, low-fat pudding, etc.)

 6. THE C GROUP: Condiments (ketchup, salad dressing, syrup, etc.) Note: Some condiments, like mustard, will be "free"—meaning they won't count in your calorie total.)

 We have also included one "T" which stands for the special antioxidant fat-burning secret tea we want you to use for this diet. See chapter 5 for the recipe!

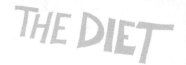

HERE'S AN EASY WAY TO REMEMBER YOUR DIET CATEGORY IN TERMS OF HEARTS, WHERE EACH HEART EQUALS ONE SERVING SIZE.

1400-CALORIE CATEGORY:

14 hearts per day (14 x 100 calories = 1400 calories)

1600-CALORIE CATEGORY:

16 hearts (16 x 100 calories = 1600 calories)

2000-CALORIE CATEGORY:

20 hearts (20 x 100 = 2000 calories)

So here it is, your diet. Look for your calorie category (either 1400, 1600, or 2000) and check out how many servings you can have from each food group. Then we'll give you a list of all the different foods you can enjoy, and we'll show you how big a serving size of each one actually is!

1400

FOOD GROUP	SERVINGS PER DAY
GRAINS, LEGUMES, OR STARCHY VEGGIES (3 SERVINGS)	♥ ♥ ♥
FRUITS (2 SERVINGS)	♥ ♥
DAIRY (2 SERVINGS)	♥ ♥
PROTEINS (2 SERVINGS)	♥ ♥
SNACKS (3 SNACKS)	♥ ♥ ♥
CONDIMENTS (1 CONDIMENT)	♥
POM TEA (1 SERVING)	♥

(Notice there are 14 hearts, with each heart representing one
100-calorie serving. Therefore 14 x 100 = 1400 calories)

1600

FOOD GROUP	SERVINGS PER DAY
GRAINS, LEGUMES, OR STARCHY VEGGIES (4 SERVINGS)	♥ ♥ ♥ ♥
FRUITS (3 SERVINGS)	♥ ♥ ♥
DAIRY (2 SERVINGS)	♥ ♥
PROTEINS (2 SERVINGS)	♥ ♥
SNACKS (3 SNACKS)	♥ ♥ ♥
CONDIMENTS (1 CONDIMENT)	♥
POM TEA (1 SERVING)	♥

(Notice there are 16 hearts, with each heart representing one 100-calorie serving. Therefore 16 x 100 = 1600 calories)

2000

FOOD GROUP	SERVINGS PER DAY
GRAINS, LEGUMES, OR STARCHY VEGGIES (5 SERVINGS)	♥ ♥ ♥ ♥ ♥
FRUITS (3 SERVINGS)	♥ ♥ ♥
DAIRY (3 SERVINGS)	♥ ♥ ♥
PROTEINS (4 SERVINGS)	♥ ♥ ♥ ♥
SNACKS (3 SNACKS)	♥ ♥ ♥
CONDIMENTS (1 CONDIMENT)	♥
POM TEA (1 SERVING)	♥

(Notice there are 20 hearts, with each heart representing one 100-calorie serving. Therefore 20 x 100 = 2000 calories)

Now you need to know the amounts and different types of foods that are in each group. So here are the lists. Keep referring back to them so that you can become fluent in the language of dieting and nutrition. It takes a while to "digest" all of this information!

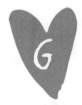

REAL SERVING SIZES OF GRAINS, LEGUMES, AND STARCHY VEGETABLES
(EACH SERVING SIZE EQUALS 100 CALORIES)

SINGLE SERVINGS OF GRAINS

- 1 English muffin

- 1 slice of rye, whole grain bread

- $1/2$ bagel

- 2 small corn tortillas

- 1 whole wheat 9" tortilla

- $1/2$ whole wheat 9" pita

♥ 2 plain breadsticks

♥ ³/₄ cup cold cereal

♥ ¹/₃ cup granola

♥ ³/₄ cup oatmeal

♥ 1 whole grain bun

♥ 2 whole grain waffles

¹/₂ CUP OF:

♥ cooked whole grain pasta

♥ brown rice

♥ wild rice

♥ basmati rice

SINGLE SERVINGS OF LEGUMES

¹/₂ CUP OF:

♥ beans

♥ lentils

56

♥ unpeeled edamame (fresh soybeans)

♥ couscous (Middle Eastern grain)

SINGLE SERVINGS OF STARCHY VEGGIES

♥ ½ cup corn, peas, or carrots

♥ 1 small yam or potato

♥ 1 vegetable roll (sushi)

♥ 1 small tomato

♥ 1 cup squash or beets

FREE NONSTARCHY VEGGIES
("FREE" MEANS YOU CAN EAT ALL YOU WANT BECAUSE THESE FOODS DON'T COUNT IN YOUR CALORIE TOTAL!)

♥ celery

♥ cucumbers

♥ green vegetables

♥ salad

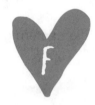

REAL SERVING SIZES OF FRUIT

(EACH SERVING SIZE EQUALS 100 CALORIES)

SINGLE SERVINGS OF FRESH FRUIT

- 1 small apple, orange, peach, plum, kiwi, tangerine, pear, nectarine, or apricot

- 1 cup pineapple, strawberries, blueberries, raspberries, or canned Mandarin oranges (unsweetented, drained)

- ¼ of a whole papaya or mango

SINGLE SERVINGS OF DRIED FRUIT

1 OUNCE (SMALL HANDFUL) OF:

- raisins

- cranberries

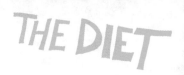

- ♥ apricots

- ♥ apples

- ♥ nectarines

- ♥ peaches

SINGLE SERVINGS OF FRUIT JUICE

6 OUNCES (SMALL JUICE GLASS) OF:

- ♥ orange juice

- ♥ apple juice

- ♥ cranberry juice

- ♥ grapefruit juice

REAL SERVING SIZES OF DAIRY

(EACH SERVING SIZE EQUALS 100 CALORIES)

SINGLE SERVINGS OF CHEESE

1.5 OUNCES (A PIECE ABOUT THE SIZE OF THREE MATCHBOXES) OF NON- OR LOW-FAT:

- cheddar

- mozzarella

- muenster

- Swiss

- string cheese

- soy cheese

- feta cheese

♥ **goat cheese**

♥ **provolone**

♥ **Asiago**

SINGLE SERVINGS OF OTHER DAIRY PRODUCTS

8 OUNCES OF:

♥ **non- or low-fat milk**

♥ **non- or low-fat soy milk**

♥ **nonfat plain yogurt**

♥ **nonfat cottage cheese**

♥ **nonfat ricotta cheese**

REAL SERVING SIZES OF PROTEINS

(EACH SERVING SIZE EQUALS 100 CALORIES)

SINGLE SERVINGS OF MEAT

3 OUNCES (ABOUT THE SIZE OF YOUR PALM) OF:

- beef (flank, round, sirloin, tenderloin, or 7 percent fat ground beef)

- skinless chicken breast (or ground chicken)

- skinless turkey breast (or ground turkey)

- pork (lean ham, tenderloin, or Canadian bacon)

- veggie or soy burger (see vegetarian alternatives)

SINGLE SERVINGS OF EGG WHITES

- 4 egg whites (1400-calorie category)

- 6 egg whites (1600-calorie category)

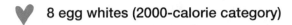 8 egg whites (2000-calorie category)

(If you love whole eggs, eat no more than 2 per week since they're high in saturated fat and cholesterol.)

SINGLE SERVINGS OF FISH

5 OUNCES (A LITTLE BIGGER THAN YOUR PALM) OF:

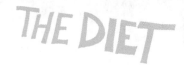 salmon

halibut

sea bass

whitefish

cod

canned tuna in water

shrimp

crab

lobster

sashimi (2 pieces for 1400-calorie diet; 2 pieces for 1600-calorie diet; 4 pieces for 2000-calorie diet)

REAL SERVING SIZES OF SNACKS

(EACH SERVING SIZE EQUALS 100 CALORIES)

SINGLE SERVINGS OF STARCHY SNACKS

- ♥ 1 ounce (about 10) whole grain crackers

- ♥ 1 ounce (about a handful) pretzels, soy chips, light cheese puffs

- ♥ 3 cups air popped popcorn

- ♥ 4 tablespoons hummus with veggies

- ♥ granola bar

SINGLE SERVINGS OF PROTEIN SNACKS

- ♥ a small 1-ounce bag turkey jerky

- ♥ 1 tablespoon peanut butter

- 1 ounce (half a handful) nuts or seeds
- 1 ounce (half a handful) chocolate-covered soy nuts
- 1 ounce Zen Mix (see recipe in chapter 5)
- Pria bar

SINGLE SERVINGS OF DAIRY SNACKS

- 4 ounce (small container) pudding
- 4 ounce (small container) low-fat frozen yogurt
- 1 Fudgsicle
- 1 low-fat string cheese
- 4 ounce Chocolate Creme (see recipe in chapter 5)
- 8 ounce nonfat latte

SINGLE SERVINGS OF FRUIT SNACKS

- 1 whole piece fresh fruit
- 1 ounce (about half your palm) dried fruit
- 1 cup canned fruit (drained, unsweetened)
- 1 frozen fruit bar, unsweetened

REAL SERVING SIZES OF CONDIMENTS

(EACH SERVING EQUALS 100 CALORIES)

SERVINGS OF CONDIMENTS

(ONE TABLESPOON OF ANY OF THE FOLLOWING EQUALS ABOUT 25 CALORIES, SO 4 TABLESPOONS = 100 CALORIES. YOU CAN USE YOUR 4 TABLESPOONS ANY WAY YOU WANT.)

- barbecue sauce

- fat-free salad dressing

- ketchup

- cocktail sauce

- relish

- low-fat sour cream

- ♥ nonfat Parmesan cheese

- ♥ low-fat mayonnaise (or the brand Lemonaise)

- ♥ salsa

- ♥ honey

- ♥ maple syrup

- ♥ pure fruit jam

OTHER CONDIMENTS

- ♥ ¼ of a small avocado

- ♥ 10 small olives

- ♥ 1 medium-size pickle

"FREE" CONDIMENTS
("FREE" MEANS YOU CAN EAT ALL YOU WANT BECAUSE THESE FOODS DON'T COUNT IN YOUR CALORIE TOTAL!)

- ♥ hot sauce

- ♥ lemon/lime juice

♥ mustard

♥ low-sodium soy sauce

♥ low-fat broth

♥ Worcestershire sauce

♥ all varieties of vinegar

"FREE" SEASONINGS
(USE AS YOU LIKE TO FLAVOR FOOD)

♥ Spike seasoning (buy at grocery story)

♥ garlic powder

♥ onion powder

♥ spices

WHAT SERVING SIZES REALLY LOOK LIKE

Now that you have the basic idea of the diet, we need to really emphasize how important it is to stick to real serving sizes, not the ones you're usually served. Here's why: super sizing is a food marketing trend in our culture that has created serving sizes that are way too big and unhealthy. Understanding healthy serving sizes is critical to your diet and your eating style in general.

In fact, a recent study done in Los Angeles backs this up. Researchers surveyed tenth grade boys and girls and found that over 60 percent of them had tried to lose weight on various diets. Who had the best results? Surprise! Not the ones who counted carbs or fat grams, but *the ones who focused on smaller serving sizes!!*

To make it easier to visualize serving sizes, we have some "show-and-tell" life-size samples [see insert]. Notice that a serving size of macaroni and cheese is about 1 cup, not the whole box. And one serving of grapes is about 15 individual grapes, not a whole bunch.

Compare the real serving size of the burger, the chicken, and the fish to what you'd be served in a restaurant. Pretty different, eh? The pizza slice is probably a lot smaller than what you'd get at a mall restaurant. One serving of cheese is really only about the size of a small toy car. Compare the muffin size to what you see in a coffee shop like Starbucks. No comparison!

Burn these images into your brain, so that when you go out to eat or when you're cooking, you'll know instinctively what one serving size is.

Now that you have your food lists and know what a serving size really is, it's time to learn how to mix and match your foods. You can't eat just anything—like 20 slices of bread in one day to fill your 20-heart allotment if you're in the 2000-calorie category. You need to eat the right number of servings from different food groups each day. Be sure you get the right amount of "hearts" from each food group: 14 total for the 1400-calorie cat-

SERVING-SIZE TIPS

 TAKE ½ CUP OF CEREAL AND PUT IT IN AN APPROPRIATELY SIZED BOWL (NOT A SOUP BOWL!). MEMORIZE WHAT IT LOOKS LIKE AND USE THAT BOWL AGAIN SO YOU CAN VISUALLY KEEP TRACK OF A SERVING SIZE. SAME GOES FOR JUICE. IF YOUR SERVING SIZE IS A CUP, NOTICE THE LEVEL OF THE JUICE IN YOUR GLASS. YOU'LL NEVER HAVE TO MEASURE AGAIN!

 BEWARE OF THE PASTA BOX! MOST PEOPLE THINK HALF A BOX IS A SERVING. IT'S NOT. A BOX USUALLY FEEDS EIGHT PEOPLE. MEASURE OUT WHAT YOU NEED AND REMEMBER THIS FORMULA: 2 OUNCES (ABOUT HALF A HANDFUL) OF DRY PASTA = 1 CUP OF COOKED PASTA.

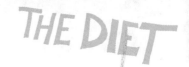

egory, 16 for the 1600-calorie category, and 20 for the 2000-calorie category. That's how you can make sure you're getting the right nutrition mix in your diet.

Here's an example. Say you are in the 1400-calorie category. Refer back to your 1400-calorie guide and pick foods from the lists of Real Serving Sizes earlier in this chapter. You'll see that you should eat the following servings of food each day (we've picked some sample foods for you here, to give you an idea):

 3 grains = muffin, 2 slices of bread

 2 fruits = banana, apple

 2 dairy = nonfat milk, cottage cheese

 2 proteins = low-fat lunch meat, grilled chicken breast

 3 snacks = Fudgsicle, string cheese, Zen Mix

 1 condiment = salad dressing

 1 Pom Tea

Now create your own menu.

BREAKFAST

MUFFIN, BANANA, COTTAGE CHEESE

LUNCH

LEAN HAM SANDWICH AND APPLE

DINNER

GRILLED CHICKEN BREAST

BIG GREEN SALAD WITH SALAD DRESSING

MILK

**Enjoy snacks and tea throughout the day,
and don't forget your "free" green veggies.*

Let's do the same mix and match for the 1600-calorie category. Refer back to your 1600-calorie Real Serving Sizes guide. Here are the amounts and kinds of foods you could pick for the day.

 4 grains = 2 pieces of whole wheat bread, cereal, wild rice

 3 fruits = strawberries, orange, blueberries

 2 dairy = nonfat milk, low-fat cheese stick

12

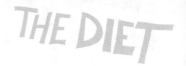

 2 proteins = 2 thin roasted turkey slices, handful of shrimp

 3 snacks = Zen Mix, peanut butter and celery, Fudgsicle

 1 condiment = cocktail sauce

 1 Pom tea

Now create your own menu.

BREAKFAST

CEREAL WITH MILK AND BLUEBERRIES

LUNCH

ROAST TURKEY SANDWICH WITH MUSTARD AND CHEESE STICK

ORANGE

DINNER

SHRIMP WITH COCKTAIL SAUCE, WILD RICE
STEAMED GREEN BEANS

STAWBERRIES

*Enjoy snacks and tea throughout the day,
and don't forget your "free" green veggies.*

Finally, let's do the same mix and match for the 2000-calorie category. Refer back to your 2000-calorie Real Serving Sizes guide. Here are the amounts and kinds of foods you could pick for the day.

- ⭐ 5 grains = a whole wheat bagel, 1 cup of cooked whole grain pasta, peas

- ⭐ 3 fruits = canned Mandarin oranges, papaya, a banana

- ⭐ 3 dairy = nonfat milk, low-fat cottage cheese, low-fat mozzarella

- ⭐ 4 proteins = a medium-size (6-ounce) chicken breast, 2 servings (or one small can) tuna in water

- ⭐ 3 snacks = Zen Mix, Chocolate Creme (see recipes in chapter 5), some watermelon

- ⭐ 1 condiment = 1/4 cup of pasta sauce

- ⭐ Pom Tea

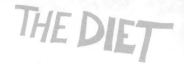

Now create your own menu.

BREAKFAST
BAGEL, PAPAYA, GLASS OF MILK

LUNCH
COTTAGE CHEESE MIXED WITH BANANA AND MANDARIN ORANGES
TUNA

DINNER
GRILLED CHICKEN BREAST, TOPPED WITH PASTA SAUCE AND MOZZARELLA
PASTA AND PEAS

**Enjoy remaining snacks and tea throughout the day,
and don't forget your "free" green veggies.*

This is your chance to design your diet every day! Now, for those of you who would like more structure and detail, the following 7-day meal plans are designed just for you! They may seem a little daunting at first, but we've included lots of cooking techniques and recipes in the next chapter, so you'll be able to follow the plans and learn a lot in the process!

1400-CALORIE 7-DAY MEAL PLAN

DAY 1

BREAKFAST

SUPER SMOOTHIE*

2 fruits, 1 dairy

LUNCH

TURKEY BURGER* ON HALF A BUN WITH LETTUCE, DIJON MUSTARD

1 protein, 1 grain, free veggies, free condiment

DINNER

BAKED ZITI WITH MEAT SAUCE AND PARMESAN CHEESE,*
MIXED GREEN SALAD WITH DRESSING

1 protein, 2 grains, 1 dairy, free veggies, 1 condiment

SNACKS

MIXED BERRIES,
ZEN MIX*, FROZEN YOGURT

1 fruit, 1 protein, 1 dairy

* = RECIPE IN CHAPTER 5

DAY 2

BREAKFAST

GRANOLA BAR,
MILK, CANTALOUPE

1 grain, 1 dairy, 1 fruit

LUNCH

CHINESE CHICKEN SALAD (GRILLED CHICKEN, LETTUCE, SLIVERED ALMONDS,
MANDARIN ORANGES WITH POPPYSEED DRESSING*), RICE CRACKERS,
COTTAGE CHEESE

1 protein, 1 grain, 1 dairy, 1 fruit, free veggies, 1 condiment

DINNER

MISO SOUP, SASHIMI AND VEGETARIAN ROLL, CUCUMBER SALAD

1 protein, 1 grain, free veggies, free condiment

SNACKS

ALMONDS, PRIA BAR, NONFAT LATTE

1 protein, 1 protein, 1 dairy

DAY 3

BREAKFAST

WHOLE GRAIN CEREAL

WITH NONFAT OR LOW-FAT SOY OR REGULAR MILK, FRESH STRAWBERRIES

1 grain, 1 dairy, 1 fruit

LUNCH

HAM AND SWISS MELT ON RYE, V-8 SOUP*, MIXED MELON CUP

1 protein, 1 grain, 1 dairy, 1 fruit, free veggies, free condiment

DINNER

GRILLED SALMON WITH LOW-FAT LEMONAISE, WILD RICE, GREEN BEANS

1 protein, 1 grain, free veggies, 1 condiment

SNACKS

PEANUT BUTTER WITH CELERY, PUDDING, CHERRIES

1 protein, 1 dairy, 1 fruit

DAY 4

BREAKFAST

WHOLE GRAIN ENGLISH MUFFIN WITH
MELTED MOZZARELLA CHEESE, MANGO

1 grain, 1 dairy, 1 fruit

LUNCH

GREEK PITA SANDWICH (PITA, CHICKEN, FETA,
ROMAINE LETTUCE, RED ONION), NECTARINE

1 protein, 1 grain 1 dairy, 1 fruit, free veggies

DINNER

OVEN-FRIED CHICKEN BREASTS* WITH APRICOT SAUCE*,
YAM FRIES*, BROCCOLI

1 protein, 1 grain, free veggies, 1 condiment

SNACKS

CASHEWS, APPLE, HUMMUS* WITH VEGGIES

1 protein, 1 fruit, 1 starch

DAY 5

BREAKFAST

EGG WHITE SCRAMBLED WITH VEGGIES,
WHOLE WHEAT TOAST, HONEYDEW MELON

1 protein, 1 grain, 1 fruit, free veggies

LUNCH

PIZZA WITH CHOICE OF VEGETABLE, MIXED GREEN SALAD, PEACH

1 grain, 1 dairy, 1 fruit, free veggies, free condiment

DINNER

LIME-CILANTRO FISH TACOS* WITH SOFT CORN TORTILLA,
JACK CHEESE, SALSA, LETTUCE

1 protein, 1 grain, 1 dairy, free veggies, 1 condiment

SNACKS

FROZEN FRUIT BAR, CHOCOLATE-COVERED SOY NUTS, TURKEY JERKY

1 fruit, 1 protein, 1 protein

DAY 6

BREAKFAST

BREAKFAST MUFFIN, YOGURT, GRAPEFRUIT

1 grain, 1 dairy, 1 fruit

LUNCH

CHICKEN CAESAR SALAD (ROASTED CHICKEN, PARMESAN, ROMAINE LETTUCE, DRESSING), WHOLE GRAIN ROLL, GRAPES

1 protein, 1 dairy, 1 grain, 1 fruit, free veggie, 1 condiment

DINNER

BBQ CHICKEN WITH BAKED BEANS, ZUCCHINI

1 protein, 1 grain, free veggies, free condiment

SNACKS

PRETZELS, FUDGSICLE, PEAR

1 grain, 1 dairy, 1 fruit

DAY 7

BREAKFAST

OATMEAL WITH BANANAS AND RAISINS, NONFAT OR LOW-FAT MILK

1 grain, 1 fruit, 1 dairy

LUNCH

TURKEY ROLL-UP (WHOLE WHEAT TORTILLA, TURKEY, CHEESE, TOMATO, SPROUTS, CUCUMBER, MUSTARD), V-8 SOUP*, KIWI

1 protein, 1 grain, 1 dairy, 1 fruit, free veggies, free condiment

DINNER

SIMPLE STIR-FRY* (BROCCOLI, WATER CHESTNUTS, SNOW PEAS, MUSHROOMS, RED PEPPER) WITH PLUM HOISIN SAUCE, BROWN RICE

1 protein, 1 grain, free veggies, 1 condiment

SNACKS

CHOCOLATE CREME*, DRIED APRICOT, SOY CHIPS

1 dairy, 1 fruit, 1 grain

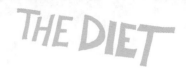

1600-CALORIE 7-DAY MEAL PLAN

DAY 1

BREAKFAST

SUPER SMOOTHIE*

2 fruits, 1 dairy

LUNCH

TURKEY BURGER* WITH BUN, LETTUCE, DIJON MUSTARD, ORANGE

1 protein, 2 grains, 1 fruit, free veggies, free condiment

DINNER

BAKED ZITI WITH MEAT SAUCE AND PARMESAN CHEESE*,
MIXED GREEN SALAD WITH DRESSING

1 protein, 2 grains, 1 dairy, free veggies, 1 condiment

SNACKS

MIXED BERRIES, ZEN MIX*, FROZEN YOGURT

1 fruit, 1 protein, 1 dairy

* = RECIPE IN CHAPTER 5

DAY 2

BREAKFAST

GRANOLA BAR, MILK, CANTALOUPE

1 grain, 1 dairy, 1 fruit

LUNCH

CHINESE CHICKEN SALAD (GRILLED CHICKEN, LETTUCE, SLIVERED ALMONDS, MANDARIN ORANGES, WITH POPPYSEED DRESSING*), RICE CRACKERS, COTTAGE CHEESE

1 protein, 1 grain, 1 dairy, 1 fruit, free veggies, 1 condiment

DINNER

EDAMAME BEANS, MISO SOUP, SASHIMI AND VEGETARIAN ROLL, CUCUMBER SALAD, ORANGE

1 protein, 1 grain, 1 starchy vegetable, 1 fruit, free veggies, free condiment

SNACKS

ALMONDS, PRIA BAR, NONFAT LATTE

1 protein, 1 protein, 1 dairy

84

CHICKEN

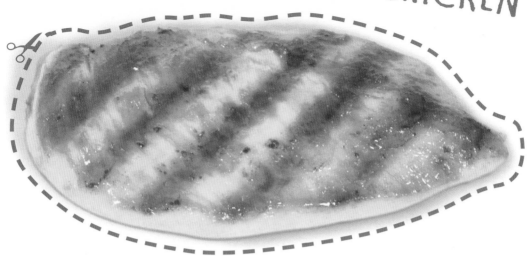

SALMON

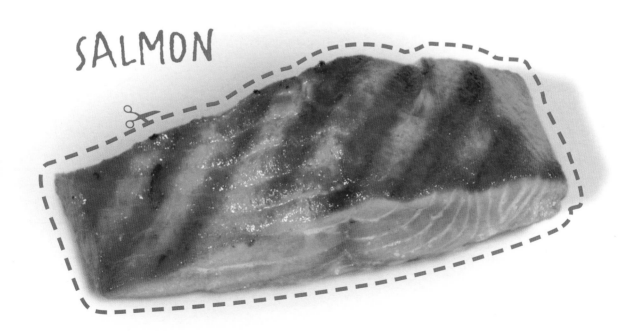

YOU MAY EXCHANGE THIS **PIECE OF CHICKEN** FOR THE SAME SERVING SIZE OF OTHER MEATS SUCH AS **PORK TENDERLOIN, LEAN STEAK,** OR **TURKEY BREAST.**

YOU MAY EXCHANGE THIS **PIECE OF SALMON** FOR THE SAME SERVING SIZE OF OTHER FISH SUCH AS **WHITEFISH, SWORDFISH,** OR **SEA BASS.**

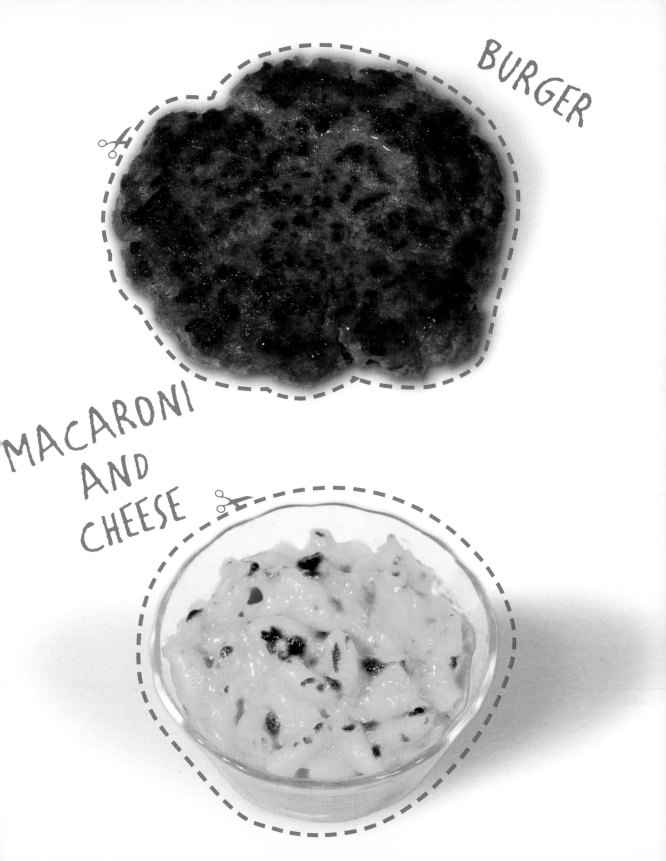

BURGER

MACARONI
AND
CHEESE

YOU MAY EXCHANGE THIS
HAMBURGER FOR THE SAME
SERVING SIZE OF TURKEY BURGER,
VEGETARIAN BURGER,
SOY BURGER,
OR LEAN BEEF BURGER.

YOU MAY EXCHANGE THIS CUP OF
MACARONI AND CHEESE FOR THE
SAME SERVING SIZE OF OTHER FOODS
SUCH AS PASTA MARINARA,
BROWN RICE,
OR LENTILS.

CHEESE PIZZA

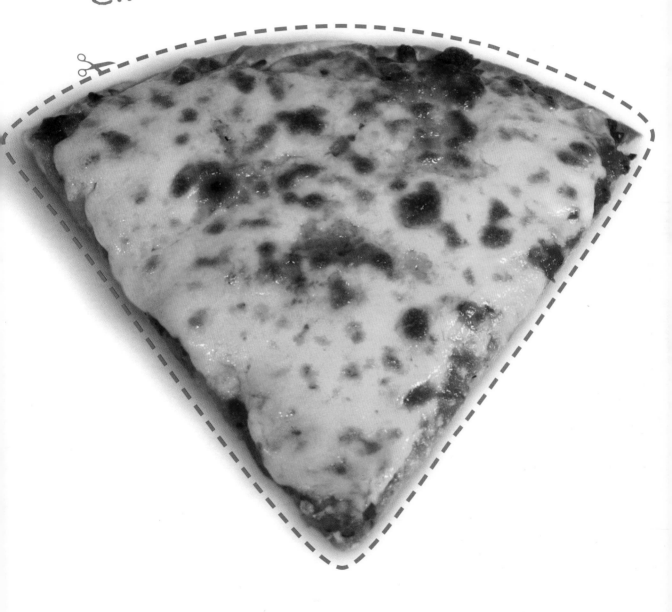

YOU MAY ENJOY THIS SERVING SIZE OF
CHEESE PIZZA WITH ANY HEALTHY TOPPING,
SUCH AS VEGETABLES,
SPINACH, OR GOAT CHEESE.

MUFFIN

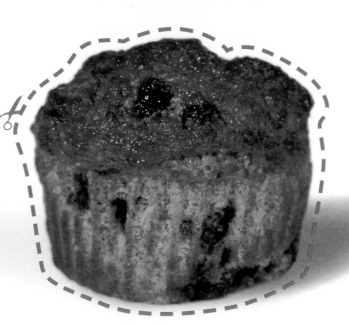

CHEESE

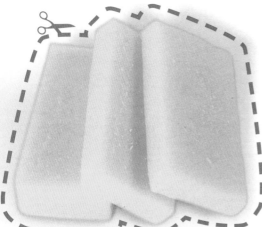

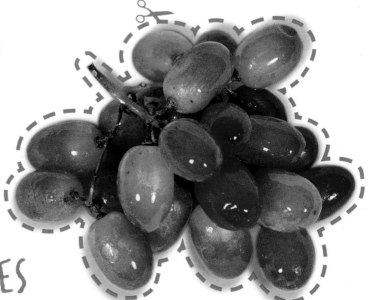

GRAPES

YOU MAY APPLY THIS SERVING SIZE TO ANY HEALTHY KIND OF **MUFFIN**, SUCH AS **STRAWBERRY, BRAN, OR APPLE.**

YOU MAY APPLY THIS SERVING SIZE TO MANY DIFFERENT KINDS OF **CHEESE**, SUCH AS **JACK, MOZZARELLA, CHEDDAR, OR SWISS.**

YOU MAY EXCHANGE THESE **GRAPES** FOR THE SAME SERVING SIZE OF OTHER **FRUITS** SUCH AS **CHERRIES** OR **MANDARIN ORANGE WEDGES.**

DAY 3

BREAKFAST

WHOLE GRAIN CEREAL WITH NONFAT OR LOW-FAT SOY OR REGULAR MILK, FRESH STRAWBERRIES

2 grains, 1 dairy, 1 fruit

LUNCH

HAM AND SWISS MELT ON RYE, V-8 SOUP*, MIXED MELON CUP

1 protein, 1 grain, 1 dairy, 1 fruit, free veggies, free condiment

DINNER

GRILLED SALMON WITH LOW-FAT LEMONAISE, WILD RICE, GREEN BEANS, TANGERINE

1 protein, 1 grain, 1 fruit, free veggies, 1 condiment

SNACKS

PEANUT BUTTER WITH CELERY, PUDDING, CHERRIES

1 protein, 1 dairy, 1 fruit

DAY 4

BREAKFAST

WHOLE GRAIN ENGLISH MUFFIN WITH MELTED MOZZARELLA, MANGO

1 fruit, 1 dairy, 1 grain

LUNCH

GREEK PITA SANDWICH (PITA, CHICKEN, FETA, ROMAINE LETTUCE, RED ONION), NECTARINE

1 protein, 2 grains, 1 dairy, 1 fruit, free veggies

DINNER

OVEN-FRIED CHICKEN BREASTS* WITH APRICOT SAUCE*, YAM FRIES*, BROCCOLI, BERRIES

1 protein, 1 grain, 1 fruit, free veggies, 1 condiment

SNACKS

CASHEWS, APPLE, HUMMUS* WITH VEGGIES

1 protein, 1 fruit, 1 protein

DAY 5

BREAKFAST

EGG WHITE SCRAMBLED WITH VEGGIES, WHOLE WHEAT TOAST, HONEYDEW MELON

1 protein, 1 grain, 1 fruit, free veggies

LUNCH

PIZZA WITH CHOICE OF VEGETABLES, MIXED GREEN SALAD, PEACH

2 grains, 1 dairy, 1 fruit, free veggies, free condiment

DINNER

LIME-CILANTRO FISH TACOS* WITH CORN TORTILLA, JACK CHEESE, SALSA, LETTUCE, PAPAYA

1 protein, 1 grain, 1 dairy, 1 fruit, free veggies, 1 condiment

SNACKS

FROZEN FRUIT BAR, CHOCOLATE-COVERED SOY NUTS, TURKEY JERKY

1 fruit, 1 protein, 1 protein

DAY 6

BREAKFAST

BREAKFAST MUFFIN, YOGURT, GRAPEFRUIT

1 grain, 1 dairy, 1 fruit

LUNCH

CHICKEN CAESAR SALAD (ROASTED CHICKEN, PARMESAN, ROMAINE LETTUCE, DRESSING), WHOLE WHEAT GRAIN ROLL, GRAPES

1 protein, 1 dairy, 1 grain, 1 fruit, free veggies, 1 condiment

DINNER

BBQ CHICKEN WITH BAKED BEANS, ZUCCHINI, WATERMELON

1 protein, 2 grains, 1 fruit, free veggies, free condiment

SNACKS

PRETZEL, FUDGSICLE, PEAR

1 grain, 1 dairy, 1 fruit

88

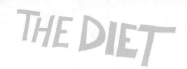

DAY 7

BREAKFAST

OATMEAL WITH BANANA AND RAISINS, NONFAT OR LOW-FAT MILK

2 grains, 1 fruit, 1 dairy

LUNCH

TURKEY ROLL-UP (WHOLE WHEAT TORTILLA, TURKEY, CHEESE, TOMATO, SPROUTS, CUCUMBER, MUSTARD), V-8 SOUP*, KIWI

1 protein, 1 grain, 1 dairy, 1 fruit, free veggies, free condiment

DINNER

SIMPLE STIR-FRY* (BROCCOLI, WATER CHESTNUTS, SNOW PEAS, MUSHROOMS, RED PEPPER) WITH PLUM HOISIN SAUCE, BROWN RICE, PEACH

1 protein, 1 grain, 1 fruit, free veggies, 1 condiment

SNACKS

CHOCOLATE CREME*, DRIED APRICOT, SOY CHIPS

1 dairy, 1 fruit, 1 grain

2000-CALORIE 7-DAY MEAL PLAN

DAY 1

BREAKFAST

SUPER SMOOTHIE*

2 fruit, 1 dairy

LUNCH

TURKEY BURGER* WITH BUN, CHEDDAR CHEESE, LETTUCE, DIJON MUSTARD, ORANGE

2 proteins, 2 grains, 1 dairy, 1 fruit, free veggies, free condiment

DINNER

BAKED ZITI WITH MEAT SAUCE AND PARMESAN CHEESE*, MIXED GREEN SALAD WITH DRESSING

2 proteins, 3 grains, 1 dairy, free veggies, 1 condiment

SNACKS

MIXED BERRIES, ZEN MIX*, FROZEN YOGURT

1 fruit, 1 protein, 1 dairy

* = RECIPE IN CHAPTER 5

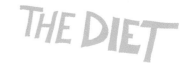

DAY 2

BREAKFAST

GRANOLA BAR, MILK, CANTALOUPE

2 grains, 1 dairy, 1 fruit

LUNCH

CHINESE CHICKEN SALAD (GRILLED CHICKEN, LETTUCE, SLIVERED ALMONDS, MANDARIN ORANGES, WITH POPPYSEED DRESSING*), RICE CRACKERS, COTTAGE CHEESE

2 proteins, 1 grains, 1 dairy, 1 fruit, free veggies, 1 condiment

DINNER

MISO SOUP, SASHIMI AND VEGETARIAN ROLL, CUCUMBER SALAD, EDAMAME BEANS, ORANGE
MILK

2 proteins, 1 grain, 1 starchy vegetable, 1 fruit, 1 dairy,
free veggies, free condiment

SNACKS

ALMONDS, PRIA BAR, NONFAT LATTE

1 protein, 1 protein, 1 dairy

DAY 3

BREAKFAST

WHOLE GRAIN CEREAL WITH NONFAT OR LOW-FAT SOY OR REGULAR MILK, FRESH STRAWBERRIES

2 grains, 1 dairy, 1 fruit

LUNCH

HAM AND SWISS MELT ON RYE, V-8 SOUP*, MILK, MIXED MELON CUP

2 proteins, 2 grains, 1 dairy, 1 fruit, 1 dairy, free veggies, free condiment

DINNER

GRILLED SALMON WITH LOW-FAT LEMONAISE, WILD RICE, GREEN BEANS, TANGERINE

2 proteins, 1 grain, 1 fruit, free veggies, 1 condiment

SNACKS

PEANUT BUTTER WITH CELERY, PUDDING, CHERRIES

1 protein, 1 dairy, 1 fruit

DAY 4

BREAKFAST

WHOLE GRAIN ENGLISH MUFFIN WITH MELTED
MOZZARELLA CHEESE, MANGO

2 grains, 1 dairy, 1 fruit

LUNCH

GREEK PITA SANDWICH (PITA, CHICKEN, FETA, ROMAINE LETTUCE,
RED ONION), NECTARINE

2 proteins, 2 grains, 1 dairy, 1 fruit, free veggies

DINNER

OVEN-FRIED CHICKEN BREASTS* WITH APRICOT SAUCE*, YAM FRIES*,
BROCCOLI AND CHEESE, BERRIES

2 proteins, 1 grain, 1 dairy, 1 fruit, free veggies, 1 condiment

SNACKS

CASHEWS, HUMMUS* WITH VEGGIES, APPLE

1 protein, 1 fruit, 1 protein

DAY 5

BREAKFAST

EGG WHITE SCRAMBLED WITH VEGGIES, WHOLE WHEAT TOAST,
HONEYDEW MELON, MILK

2 proteins, 1 grain, 1 fruit, 1 dairy, free veggies

LUNCH

PIZZA WITH CHOICE OF VEGETABLE, MIXED GREEN SALAD
WITH DRESSING, PEACH

2 grains, 1 dairy, 1 fruit, free veggies, free condiment

DINNER

LIME-CILANTRO FISH TACOS* WITH CORN TORTILLAS, JACK CHEESE,
SALSA, LETTUCE, PAPAYA

2 proteins, 2 grains, 1 dairy, 1 fruit, free veggies, 1 condiment

SNACKS

FROZEN FRUIT BAR, CHOCOLATE-COVERED SOY NUTS, TURKEY JERKY

1 fruit, 1 protein, 1 protein

94

DAY 6

BREAKFAST

BREAKFAST MUFFIN, YOGURT, GRAPEFRUIT

2 grains, 1 dairy, 1 fruit

LUNCH

CHICKEN CAESAR SALAD (ROASTED CHICKEN, PARMESAN, ROMAINE LETTUCE, DRESSING), WHOLE WHEAT GRAIN ROLL, GRAPES

2 proteins, 1 dairy, 1 grain, 1 fruit, free veggies, 1 condiment

DINNER

BBQ CHICKEN WITH BAKED BEANS, ZUCCHINI, MILK, WATERMELON

2 proteins, 2 grains, 1 dairy, 1 fruit, free veggies, free condiment

SNACKS

PRETZEL, FUDGSICLE, PEAR

1 grain, 1 dairy, 1 fruit

DAY 7

BREAKFAST

OATMEAL WITH BANANA AND RAISINS, NONFAT OR LOW-FAT MILK

2 grains, 1 fruit, 1 dairy

LUNCH

TURKEY ROLL-UP (WHOLE WHEAT TORTILLA, TURKEY, CHEESE, TOMATO, SPROUTS, CUCUMBER, MUSTARD), V-8 SOUP*, KIWI

2 proteins, 1 grain, 1 dairy, 1 fruit, free veggies, free condiment

DINNER

SIMPLE STIR-FRY* (BROCCOLI, WATER CHESTNUTS, SNOW PEAS, MUSHROOMS, RED PEPPER), WITH PLUM HOISIN SAUCE, BROWN RICE, MILK, PEACH

2 proteins, 2 grains, 1 dairy, 1 fruit, free veggies, 1 condiment

SNACKS

CHOCOLATE CREME*, DRIED APRICOT, SOY CHIPS

1 dairy, 1 fruit, 1 grain

96

VEGETARIAN ALTERNATIVES

Being a vegetarian is a matter of choice. Some people eat this way because they think it's healthier, while others do it to support animal rights. Should you eat this way? Generally speaking, now is a good time to eat all different kinds of food, and eating a vegetarian diet can be challenging if you want to achieve optimum nutritional balance. Still, you can eat a healthful and balanced diet; we offer the following information and alternatives.

There are several types of vegetarians:

★ **Lacto-ovo vegetarians eat dairy and egg products.**

★ **Lacto-vegetarians eat dairy and no eggs.**

★ **Ovo-vegetarians eat eggs and no dairy.**

★ **Vegans eat only from plant sources—no eggs, dairy, or honey.**

Most vegetarians eat more fruits and vegetables than nonvegetarians. Not a bad thing, but it may leave you deficient in certain nutrients like protein and minerals such as iron, calcium, zinc, vitamin D, and vitamin B_{12}. So the challenge is to get *adequate complete protein* (that is, all nine essential amino acids). You won't be able to get this from any plant food except soy.

Another way to get complete protein is to combine foods. If you eat legumes and grains (such as beans and rice) together, you create a complete protein. You can do the same with legumes by adding seeds or nuts. You don't need complete proteins at every meal, as long as you eat them during the course of the day.

There are also lots of prepared foods that can serve as protein substitutes. Just switch the following vegetarian foods for the meats listed in your calorie category.

VEGETARIAN PROTEIN SUBSTITUTES

ITEM	SERVING SIZE	CALORIES	PROTEIN	CARBS	FAT
VEGGIE HOT DOG	1	100	16g	7g	1.5g
VEGGIE BURGER	1 PATTY	100	8g	9g	3g
SOY BURGER	1 PATTY	100	16g	9g	4g
SOY SLICES	4	80	3g	4g	1g
SOY CHEESE	1.5 oz	100	12g	1.5g	5g
SOY MILK	8 oz	100	7g	4g	5g

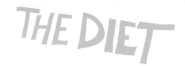

ITEM	SERVING SIZE	CALORIES	PROTEIN	CARBS	FAT
TOFU	3 oz	100	14g	4g	4g
TEMPEH	⅓ CUP	100	12g	6g	7g
SEITAN	3 oz	100	31g	3g	1g

Okay, that should cover you! Remember, all this information won't sink in after just one reading. We want you to keep coming back to this chapter to review your serving sizes and food choices, so you can learn to mix and match foods and get good at figuring out what a serving size is. Hopefully, you'll be able to use this information for the rest of your life, so you can eat the delicious foods that are best for you!

LET ME COOK!

★FIVE★

You are a lucky girl! People have been begging for the recipes that we're about to give you from Carrie's Diet Designs company because they're mouthwateringlowcaloriehighnutrientdensity foods! Until now, the recipes have been in top-secret files.

Why are you getting them? Because we love you! Also, because these are all simple recipes that will get you cooking and taking charge of your food. Save money, make your taste buds happy, and impress family and friends with your culinary skills!

First, we'll give you some basic cooking techniques that will last you a lifetime, and then we'll give you the recipes. The cooking techniques are designed to make your meals healthful, low in fat and calories, yet big on taste. Bon appétit!

LOW-FAT COOKING TECHNIQUES

SAUTÉING

DID YOU KNOW THAT COOKING WITH LIQUIDS OTHER THAN FAT CAN CUT THE FAT CONTENT OF A DISH BY UP TO 1000 CALORIES?!

Instead of using fat, like butter or oils, *use liquids*! Sautéing your food means to take something like a chicken breast and cook it in a liquid in a stovetop pan. Choose your liquid from the following list, or mix and match!

 Chicken stock

 Vegetable stock

 Fruit juice

 Vinegar

 Soy sauce

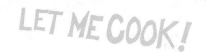

Then follow these simple steps:

1. Heat 2 tablespoons of liquid in a sauté pan over medium-high heat.

2. When the liquid begins to steam, add vegetables, meat, or poultry and stir.

3. Continue to sauté, stirring frequently, until the liquid in the pan evaporates. As soon as it evaporates, quickly add 2 more tablespoons of liquid, stirring contents to scrape up the glaze formed at the bottom of the pan.

4. Continue to sauté, adding liquid in small amounts as necessary, until done. Meats and poultry should be browned on the outside and cooked through; onions should be very soft and a caramelized brown; other vegetables should be tender.

GRILLING, BAKING, AND POACHING

Poultry, meats, and seafood all contain natural fats, and should be cooked without any additional oils except where a recipe calls for it.

1. GRILLING is the fastest cooking method, and it works best with thicker cuts. Begin with a preheated grill or broiler, and put your

meat on the grill or a few inches under the broiler, turning when the grilled side is done (fish should flake; poultry should begin to brown). Flip and cook the other side: the second side will probably require less time. Depending on thickness, grill 5 to 7 minutes per side. For extra flavor and moisture, brush seafood, meat, or poultry with fresh citrus juice, mustard, Worcestershire sauce, soy sauce, or fresh herbs before grilling or roasting. An oil-free marinade is also a great alternative; for best flavor, marinate for at least 2 hours or overnight in the refrigerator.

2. **BAKING** is a slower cooking method. Bake most cuts for 20 to 30 minutes at 350°F. The time will vary depending on what you're cooking. Cut into the middle of the meat after about 20 minutes to see if it's done enough for you.

3. **POACHING** involves a slow simmer in liquid, like water or stock or broth that can be flavored with herbs, onions, shallots (similar to an onion), or garlic. In a wide saucepan, add the food in a single layer with enough liquid to just cover the food. Heat, uncovered, to a very slow simmer for 7 to 10 minutes. For extra flavor, remove food and reduce the cooking liquid (that is, let the liquid simmer until it thickens) to 2 tablespoons. Poaching is a good choice for delicate cuts like chicken breast, fish fillets, and shellfish.

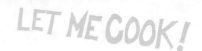

THICKENING SAUCES

1. Substitute stock or broth for butter, cooking it into a paste with a tablespoon or two of flour before whisking in hot liquid.

2. Substitute skim milk (regular or evaporated), buttermilk, or yogurt for cream. To prevent curdling (lumpiness), add 1 teaspoon corn-starch per cup of liquid.

3. Finish sauces with arrowroot (looks like flour) instead of butter by dissolving about 1 tablespoon of arrowroot per cup of sauce in cold stock, milk, or water. Whisk into sauce and cook over low to medium heat until you get the desired consistency.

SALAD DRESSING

Eliminate oil, mayonnaise, and sour cream in general; mix and match from the following ingredients:

1. **Vinegar (all types and flavors)**

2. **Mustard (all types and flavors)**

3. **Fruit juices and concentrates**

4. **Fresh and dried herbs and spices**

5. **Garlic, onions, and shallots**

6. **Chicken or vegetable stock**

7. **Honey**

8. **Fat-free mayonnaise, ricotta cheese, buttermilk**

PASTA LOVER TIPS

1. Always select pasta made without oils or eggs, and try to get whole grain pasta whenever you can.

2. Many pasta boxes instruct you to add oil and salt to the cooking water. There's no need for the extra fat and sodium; your sauce will provide plenty of flavor and moisture.

3. Pasta should always be cooked in a large pot of boiling water. Add pasta to the pot gradually so that the water continues to boil.

4. 2 ounces of dry pasta is about the width of a quarter and yields 1 to 1½ cups cooked, depending on the type.

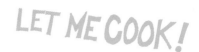

MEASURING TIPS

You'll notice that there are wet and dry weight measures. Though ounces are used for both weight and liquid volume, they are not equivalent! And while the amounts in wet and dry measuring cups are the same, each type is designed for more accurate measuring of the contents.

Here's the breakdown.

1 cup = 8 fluid ounces

³/₄ cup = 6 fluid ounces

¹/₂ cup = 4 fluid ounces

¹/₄ cup = 2 fluid ounces

1 pound = 16 ounces by weight

³/₄ pound = 12 ounces by weight

¹/₂ pound = 8 ounces by weight

¹/₄ pound = 4 ounces by weight

Here are some conversions.

3 teaspoons = 1 tablespoon

2 tablespoons = ¹/₈ cup

4 tablespoons = $\frac{1}{4}$ cup

8 tablespoons = $\frac{1}{2}$ cup

16 tablespoons = 1 cup

1 pint = 2 cups

1 quart = 4 cups

HUNGRY? GREAT, IT'S TIME TO COOK! HERE ARE THE RECIPES!

EASIEST BANANA-BUTTER WAFFLES EVER

1. Toast a frozen whole grain waffle.

2. Mash a banana with a fork until it's goopy.

3. Spread the banana on the waffle like butter. Enjoy!

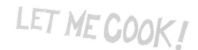

MAGIC LOW-FAT STRAWBERRY-CINNAMON MUFFINS

MAKES 12 MUFFINS

Cooking spray

1 1/2 cups whole wheat flour

1/2 cup plus 1 tablespoon packed brown sugar

2 1/2 teaspoons baking powder

1 1/2 teaspoons ground cinnamon

1/4 teaspoon salt

2/3 cup nonfat vanilla yogurt

1/4 cup margarine, melted

3 tablespoons 1-percent low-fat milk

1 large egg, lightly beaten

1/4 cup pure fruit strawberry jam, no sugar added

1. Preheat the oven to 375°F. Put a muffin liner into each cup of a 12-cup muffin pan, coat the liners with cooking spray.

2. Lightly spoon the flour into dry measuring cups, and level with a knife. In a large bowl, combine the flour, 1/2 cup of the brown sugar, baking powder, 1 teaspoon of the cinnamon, and salt, whisking well.

3. In a small bowl, combine the yogurt, margarine, milk, and egg, whisking well.

4. Make a well in the center of the flour mixture. Add the yogurt mixture to the flour mixture, stirring just until moist.

5. Spoon 1 tablespoon of batter into each liner. Top the batter with 1 teaspoon jam. Top evenly with the remaining batter.

6. Combine the remaining 1 tablespoon brown sugar and ¹/₂ teaspoon cinnamon; sprinkle over the batter. Bake for 20 to 25 minutes, until lightly brown on top.

7. Remove the muffins from the pan and place on a wire rack to cool.

SUPER SMOOTHIE

MAKES 1 SMOOTHIE

$1/2$ cup unfiltered apple juice

$1/4$ cup ice

$1/2$ cup plain, nonfat yogurt

$1/2$ cup cubed papaya

$1/2$ cup sliced strawberries

1 tablespoon toasted wheat germ

$1/2$ scoop whey protein powder

Mix all the ingredients in a blender until smooth (about a minute).

Pour and enjoy!

OVEN-FRIED CHICKEN BREASTS

MAKES 4 SERVINGS

Cooking spray

$\frac{1}{4}$ cup dry bread crumbs

2 tablespoons grated Parmesan cheese

1 teaspoon paprika

1 teaspoon dried thyme

$\frac{1}{2}$ teaspoon garlic salt

$\frac{1}{4}$ teaspoon ground red pepper

$\frac{1}{2}$ cup low-fat buttermilk

1 pound boneless, skinless chicken breasts

1 tablespoon margarine, melted

1. Preheat the oven to 400°F. Coat a shallow baking dish with the cooking spray.

2. In a separate shallow bowl, combine the bread crumbs, cheese, paprika, thyme, salt, and red pepper.

3. Place buttermilk in another shallow dish. Dip the chicken in the buttermilk.

112

4. Now dip the chicken in the bread crumb mixture so it is lightly coated.

5. Place the chicken, rounded sides up, in the shallow baking dish and drizzle the margarine over the chicken.

6. Bake for 40 minutes, or until browned. We recommend serving this dish with the apricot sauce (see next recipe).

APRICOT SAUCE

MAKES 8 SERVINGS

$1/3$ **cup apricot preserves**

$1/8$ **cup Dijon mustard**

$1/4$ **cup low-sodium soy sauce**

In a small bowl, blend all ingredients with a wire whisk for several minutes. Serve chilled or warm with oven-fried chicken or any other poultry or seafood.

LIME-CILANTRO FISH TACOS

MAKES 4 SERVINGS

2 teaspoons olive oil

1 pound halibut, red snapper, or any whitefish trimmed and cut into thin strips

$1/4$ teaspoon salt

$1/8$ teaspoon freshly ground black pepper

$1/2$ cup sliced fresh mango

$1 1/2$ cups thinly sliced onions

1 small jalapeño pepper, seeded and chopped (or canned)

$1/2$ cup fat-free, low-sodium chicken broth

$1/2$ cup chopped plum tomatoes

3 tablespoons chopped fresh cilantro

$2 1/2$ tablespoons fresh lime juice

8 (6-inch) flour tortillas

1. Heat a large nonstick skillet over medium-high heat with the oil.

2. Season the fish with salt and black pepper.

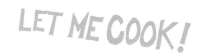

3. Place the fish in the pan, and sauté for 4 minutes, or until browned. Remove the fish from the pan; place in a bowl.

4. Add the mango, onions, and jalapeño to the pan; sauté for 5 minutes, or until tender.

5. Add the broth, reduce the heat, and simmer 1 minute, scraping the pan to loosen browned bits. Stir in the tomatoes; simmer for 2 minutes.

6. Return the fish and the accumulated juices to the pan. Stir in the cilantro and lime juice; cook 1 minute, or until fish is done (it will be opaque and flaky).

7. Heat the tortillas according to the package directions. Spoon $1/2$ cup of fish mixture onto each tortilla; roll them up and serve.

TURKEY BURGERS

MAKES 4 SERVINGS

1 pound ground turkey breast

$\frac{1}{2}$ cup sourdough bread crumbs

$\frac{1}{4}$ cup low-fat buttermilk

$\frac{1}{4}$ cup minced green onion

$\frac{1}{4}$ cup chopped parsley

$\frac{1}{2}$ teaspoon Dijon mustard

$\frac{1}{2}$ teaspoon Worcestershire sauce

Dash of black pepper

1. In a large bowl, combine all the ingredients. Divide the mixture into 4 equal portions and form into patties.

2. Grill or broil the burgers for 15 minutes, until browned and cooked thoroughly.

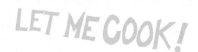

BAKED ZITI WITH MEAT SAUCE AND PARMESAN CHEESE

MAKES 8 SERVINGS

Cooking spray

16 ounces whole wheat ziti

1 pound turkey sausage

1 cup chopped onion

2 cloves garlic, minced

24 ounces marinara sauce

$1/4$ teaspoon salt

$1/4$ teaspoon black pepper

1 tablespoon Italian seasoning

2 cups shredded mozzarella cheese

1 cup grated Parmesan cheese

1. Preheat the oven to 350°F.

2. Cook the pasta according to the package directions, omitting the salt and oil. Drain the pasta and set aside.

3. Remove the sausage casings. Cook the sausage, onion, and garlic in a large nonstick skillet over medium heat until browned, stirring to crumble.

4. Add the marinara sauce, salt, pepper, and Italian seasoning, and bring to a boil. Cover, reduce heat, and simmer 10 minutes, stirring occasionally.

5. Combine the cooked pasta and sausage mixture. Place half of the pasta mixture in a 4-quart casserole dish coated with cooking spray. Top with half of the mozzarella and half of the Parmesan. Repeat the layers. Bake for 25 minutes or until the cheese is bubbly.

6. Let the baked ziti cool for a few minutes and cut into 8 servings.

SIMPLE STIR-FRY

MAKES 3 SERVINGS (4 CUPS)

9 ounces firm low-fat tofu, cut into 1-inch pieces

2 tablespoons bottled hoisin sauce

1 teaspoon sesame oil

1 teaspoon low-sodium soy sauce

1 teaspoon minced garlic

1 teaspoon minced ginger

$1/4$ cup chopped scallions

$1/4$ whole yellow bell pepper, thinly sliced

2 medium carrots, cut in $1/2$-inch pieces

1 cup snow peas

1 cup chopped broccoli

4 ounces canned water chestnuts, drained

1 14-ounce can chicken or vegetable broth (optional)

1. Place the tofu cubes in a small bowl and marinate in the hoisin sauce. In a large sauté pan or wok, place the sesame oil, soy sauce, garlic, and ginger. Stir-fry on medium heat for several minutes and then add the scallions, pepper, and carrots.

2. Continue stirring for 5 more minutes. Add the snow peas, broccoli, and water chestnuts, and stir for several minutes (add more soy sauce and chicken broth if needed).

3. Finally, add the marinated tofu to the vegetable mixture and cook thoroughly for 5 minutes, or until browned.

MACARONI AND CHEESE

MAKES 9 SERVINGS (4 CUPS)

- 1 tablespoon margarine
- 2 tablespoons all-purpose flour
- 1 $\frac{1}{4}$ cups skim milk
- 1 $\frac{1}{2}$ cups shredded reduced-fat sharp cheddar cheese
- 3 tablespoons grated low-fat Parmesan cheese
- 1 teaspoon low-sodium Worcestershire sauce
- $\frac{1}{2}$ teaspoon dry mustard
- $\frac{1}{8}$ teaspoon pepper
- $\frac{1}{8}$ teaspoon hot sauce (optional)
- 4 cups cooked elbow macaroni

1. Melt the margarine in a saucepan over medium heat, then add the flour. Cook 1 minute, stirring constantly with a wire whisk. Gradually add the milk while stirring.

2. Bring to a boil. Cook 1 minute, stirring constantly.

3. Remove the pan from the heat. Add the cheeses, Worcestershire sauce, mustard, pepper, and hot sauce (if using), stirring until the

cheese melts. In a large bowl, combine the cheese sauce and macaroni; stir well.

4. Serve immediately.

QUICKEST TUNA SALAD

MAKES 2 SERVINGS (1 CUP)

7 $\frac{1}{2}$ ounces canned tuna in water, drained

1 tablespoon Lemonaise, light or Best Foods Light

Mixed greens or whole grain bread

1. In a small bowl, mix together the tuna and Lemonaise.

2. Place the tuna on mixed greens or bread.

V-8 SOUP

MAKES 12 SERVINGS

3 quarts V-8 vegetable juice, no added salt

2 cans low-fat, low-sodium chicken broth

1 medium onion, quartered

2 stalks celery, cut up

3 cups chopped broccoli

2 cups string beans

2 cups cut-up zucchini

10 ounces frozen peas

1 tablespoon dry or fresh thyme

1 tablespoon dry or fresh basil

1. Place V-8 juice, chicken broth, and onion in a large stockpot. Cook on medium heat for approximately 10 minutes, stirring occasionally.

2. Add the remaining vegetables and simmer for an additional 15 minutes, or until vegetables are cooked through. Add seasonings, stir, and serve.

YAM FRIES

MAKES 2 SERVINGS

Cooking spray

2 pounds yams, cut into $1/2$-inch sticks

2 tablespoons frozen orange juice concentrate, thawed

1 teaspoon onion powder (optional)

$1/2$ teaspoon salt (optional)

$1/8$ teaspoon ground red pepper (optional)

1. Preheat oven to 375°F. Line cookie sheet with foil and spray with cooking spray.

2. In a medium bowl, season the yam sticks with the orange juice concentrate, and if desired, onion powder, salt, and pepper.

3. Place single layer of the yams onto the cookie sheet. Bake for 10 minutes, or until side is browned; turn once, bake for 10 more minutes, or until yams are crisp.

HUMMUS

MAKES 8 SERVINGS

1 pound garbanzo beans, canned and drained

1 $\frac{1}{2}$ tablespoons plain, nonfat yogurt

2 teaspoons minced garlic

2 tablespoons fresh lemon juice

$\frac{3}{4}$ teaspoon chopped fresh parsley

1 dash cayenne pepper

Salt to taste

1. Combine all of the ingredients in a food processor and process until smooth.

2. Chill in the refrigerator for at least 1 hour, and serve.

SUPER SIMPLE CHEESE "CHIPS"

MAKES 8 SERVINGS

1 block (14 ounces) low-fat cheddar cheese (we recommend Horizon organic)

1. Cut domino-size pieces from the block of cheese.

2. Place the cheese on a nonstick pan over medium to low heat. Cook until the cheese melts and starts to crisp.

3. Flip the pieces over, crisp the other side, and let cool on a paper towel.

ZEN MIX

MAKES 8 SERVINGS

$\frac{1}{2}$ cup dried cranberries

$\frac{1}{4}$ cup roasted shelled sunflower seeds

$\frac{1}{4}$ cup dry-roasted soy nuts

$\frac{1}{4}$ cup raw pepitas (shelled pumpkin seeds)

Mix all ingredients in a bowl and serve.

POPPYSEED DRESSING

MAKES 8 SERVINGS

1 cup frozen apple juice concentrate, thawed

6 tablespoons fresh lemon juice

6 tablespoons balsamic vinegar

4 tablespoons Dijon mustard

2 tablespoons honey

1 tablespoon poppyseeds

1 teaspoon black pepper

Whisk together all ingredients in a small bowl. Cover and refrigerate. Serve chilled on any fresh salad.

CHOCOLATE CREME DESSERT

MAKES 4 SERVINGS

2 ounces light cream cheese

1 tablespoon powdered fructose

2 teaspoons unsweetened cocoa powder

15 ounces fat-free ricotta cheese

$1/2$ cup fresh raspberries

1. In a medium bowl, blend together the cream cheese, fructose, and the cocoa on medium speed for 1 minute or until smooth. Scrape the bowl and add the ricotta cheese.

2. Whip with a wire whisk to remove the lumps. Mix for another minute to fully blend. Chill for 1 hour.

3. Serve with raspberries on top.

CHOCOLATE CHIP BARS

MAKES 24 SERVINGS

Cooking spray

1 $\frac{1}{3}$ **cups all-purpose flour**

1 teaspoon baking powder

1 teaspoon salt

4 tablespoons reduced-calorie margarine

$\frac{1}{4}$ **cup nonfat cream cheese**

1 cup packed light brown sugar

1 cup granulated sugar

2 large eggs

3 teaspoons vanilla

1 cup miniature chocolate chips

1. Preheat oven to 350ºF. Spray a 9 x 13-inch pan lightly with cooking spray.

2. Stir together flour, baking powder, and salt. Set aside.

3. Melt the margarine in a pan, let it cook until it turns a nutty brown color, and pour into a large mixing bowl.

4. Add the cream cheese and both brown and white sugars; beat until smooth. Add the eggs and vanilla; beat until blended.

5. Add the reserved dry ingredients and the chocolate chips, and mix until well blended.

6. Pour batter into prepared pan.

7. Bake for 15 to 20 minutes, or until golden brown.

8. Cool and cut into 4 crosswise and 6 lengthwise cuts.

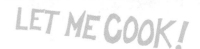

THE MOST SECRET RECIPE OF ALL

First, a little bit about this totally unique beverage. We make it by combining pure pomegranate juice and a special green tea.

The Buddhists believe that the pomegranate is one of the most blessed and sacred fruits. The health benefits include a powerful blend of antioxidants that work together to prevent certain cancers, heart disease, and premature aging. It also acts as a hormone balancer, which is essential for women—especially teenagers. The best part of this elixir is that it contains compounds that work with your metabolism to *increase fat burning*.

You can drink up to 16 ounces per day, ideally after breakfast and again in the afternoon. If you prefer it to be sweeter you can use a small amount of stevia, a natural sweetener made from chickory plant extracts that you'll find at most health food stores.

POM TEA

MAKES 5 SERVINGS

5 bags of green tea with chamomile (we use Celestial Seasonings Chamomile Green Tea)

8 ounces pure pomegranate juice (we use Pom Wonderful)

4 cups boiling water

1. Add the teabags to the boiling water. Steep (let the teabags sit in hot water) for about 5 minutes.

2. Remove the tea bags and add the pomegranate juice.

You can prepare Pom Tea ahead of time in a large batch to last you several days, or prepare it by the cup. Drink it hot or iced, but remember to take a deep breath and close your eyes when you do. It will help you burn fat *and* calm your nerves. Ohmmmmm.

Here's to the new chef in you!

LAUGHTER IS BRIGHTEST WHERE FOOD IS BEST.

—IRISH PROVERB

GROCERY SHOPPING 101 ★ SIX ★★

Shopping for your own food? Good idea! Not only will you save money, but you'll outsmart all those clever food marketers, vending machine operators, and fast-food chains who want you to buy their high-fat, high-calorie foods!

But first, have you ever looked at one of those nutrition labels on packaged foods and wondered how much fat is too much? Or how much fiber you need? Or what exactly cholesterol is, anyway? Since we have a nutritionist "in the house," we can ask.

Let's start with some label reading basics. First up: how to figure out serving *sizes* from labels. Here's one from Frosted Flakes. Pay attention to the circled number—that's how you find out how big a serving size is.

KELLOGG'S FROSTED FLAKES

Nutrition Facts

Serving Size ¾ Cup (31g/1.1 oz.)
Servings Per Container About 18

Amount Per Serving	Cereal	Cereal with ½ Cup Vitamins A & D Fat Free Milk
Calories	120	160
Calories from Fat	0	0
	%Daily Value**	
Total Fat 0g*	0%	0%
Saturated Fat 0g	0%	0%
Trans Fat 0g		
Cholesterol 0mg	0%	0%
Sodium 150mg	6%	9%
Potassium 20mg	1%	6%
Total Carbohydrate 28g	9%	11%
Dietary Fiber 1g	3%	3%
Sugars 12g		
Other Carbohydrate 15g		
Protein 1g		

NOTICE HOW ONE SERVING IS REALLY ONLY ¾ OF A CUP! THIS IS WHAT YOU'RE REALLY SUPPOSED TO HAVE, BUT MOST PEOPLE FILL THEIR BOWLS WITH 3 TIMES AS MUCH.

Now let's compare this label to another popular cereal label, Cheerios.

Check out the sugar amount:

CHEERIOS

KELLOGG'S FROSTED FLAKES

Nutrition Facts

Serving Size   ¾ Cup (31g/1.1 oz.)
Servings Per Container   About 18

Amount Per Serving	Cereal	Cereal with ½ Cup Vitamins A & D Fat Free Milk
Calories	120	160
Calories from Fat	0	0
	%Daily Value**	
Total Fat 0g*	0%	0%
Saturated Fat 0g	0%	0%
Trans Fat 0g		
Cholesterol 0mg	0%	0%
Sodium 150mg	6%	9%
Potassium 20mg	1%	6%
Total Carbohydrate 28g	9%	11%
Dietary Fiber 1g	3%	3%
Sugars 12g		
Other Carbohydrate 15g		
Protein 1g		

Nutrition Facts

Serving Size   1 Cup (30g)
         Children Under 4 – ¾ Cup (20g)
Servings Per Container   About 9
         Children Under 4 – About 14

Amount Per Serving	Cheerios	with ½ Cup skim milk	Cereal for Children Under 4
Calories	110	150	70
Calories from Fat	15	20	10
	% Daily Value**		
Total Fat 2g*	3%	3%	1g
Saturated Fat 0g	0%	3%	0g
Trans Fat 0g			0g
Polyunsaturated Fat 0.5g			0g
Monounsaturated Fat 0.5g			0g
Cholesterol 0mg	0%	1%	0mg
Sodium 210mg	9%	12%	140mg
Potassium 200mg	6%	12%	130mg
Total Carbohydrate 22g	7%	9%	15g
Dietary Fiber 3g	11%	11%	2g
Soluble Fiber 1g			0g
Sugars 1g			1g
Other Carbohydrate 18g			12g
Protein 3g			2g

THIS IS SO HIGH IN SUGAR

LOW SUGAR IS GREAT!

Now let's take a look at potato chip labels. We have regular Lay's and Baked Lay's. What's the big issue here? Fat and calories.

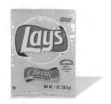

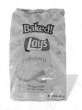

Nutrition Facts

Serving Size 1 package
Servings Per Container 1

Amount Per Serving

Calories 150	Calories from Fat 90
	% Daily Value
Total Fat 10g	**15%**
Saturated Fat 3g	**15%**
Trans Fat 0g	
Cholesterol 0mg	**0%**
Sodium 180mg	**8%**
Total Carbohydrate 15g	**5%**
Dietary Fiber 1g	**4%**
Sugars 0g	
Protein 2g	

Nutrition Facts

Serving Size 1 oz. (28g/About 11 crisps)
Servings Per Container 10

Amount Per Serving

Calories 110	Calories from Fat 15
	% Daily Value
Total Fat 1.5g	**2%**
Saturated Fat 0g	**0%**
Trans Fat 0g	
Cholesterol 0mg	**0%**
Sodium 150mg	**6%**
Total Carbohydrate 23g	**8%**
Dietary Fiber 2g	**6%**
Sugars 2g	
Protein 2g	

CLASSIC LAY'S POTATO CHIPS

10 TIMES MORE FAT THAN BAKED!
(PLUS THERE'S SATURATED FAT, WHICH
BELONGS IN ANIMALS, NOT
POTATOES!)

BAKED! LAY'S POTATO CHIPS

THIS IS A GREAT SNACK! FAT IS
BELOW 5 GRAMS, AND CALORIES ARE
LOW! (PLUS NO SATURATED FAT!)

136

Sometimes just reading a label carefully and comparing products can save you lots of fat grams. Take, for example, chicken nuggets. We're comparing the Tyson brand with a brand found in health food stores called Ian's. Our own taste tests show that Ian's chicken nuggets are delicious, so taste isn't a factor here.

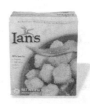

Nutrition Facts

Serving Size 5 pieces (90g)
Servings Per Container About 3.5

Amount Per Serving

Calories 280	Calories from Fat 150

	% Daily Value**
Total Fat 16g	**25%**
Saturated Fat 4g	**20%**
Cholesterol 50mg	**17%**
Sodium 430mg	**18%**
Total Carbohydrate 21g	**7%**
Dietary Fiber 0g	**0%**
Sugars 1g	
Protein 13g	**26%**

Nutrition Facts

Serving Size 3 oz. (84g) about 5 nuggets
Servings Per Container About 3

Amount Per Serving

Calories 190	Calories from Fat 70

	% Daily Value**
Total Fat 8g	**12%**
Saturated Fat 2g	**10%**
Cholesterol 40mg	**13%**
Sodium 250mg	**10%**
Total Carbohydrate 14g	**5%**
Dietary Fiber 0g	**0%**
Sugars 1g	
Protein 15g	

TYSON BREAST NUGGETS

16 GRAMS OF FAT—
WAY TOO HIGH!

IAN'S CHICKEN NUGGETS

8 GRAMS OF FAT—BETTER!
(PLUS PROTEIN IS HIGHER AND
CARBS ARE LOWER.)

Pizza seems to be a staple in just about everyone's diet, but watch out for what you'll find inside. This is a label from a frozen Celeste Pepperoni Pizza.

Nutrition Facts

Serving Size 1 pizza (158g)
Servings Per Container 1

Amount Per Serving

Calories 410   Calories from Fat 190

	% Daily Value**
Total Fat 21g	**32%**
Saturated Fat 7g	**35%**
Trans Fat 3.5g	
Polyunsaturated Fat 2.5g	
Monounsaturated Fat 7.5g	
Cholesterol 15mg	**5%**
Sodium 1190mg	**50%**
Total Carbohydrate 41g	**14%**
Dietary Fiber 4g	**12%**
Sugars 7g	
Protein 14g	

CELESTE PEPPERONI PIZZA

WOW, 21 GRAMS OF FAT! AND MUCH OF IT IS SATURATED AND TRANS FAT—NOT GOOD! PLUS THAT'S A LOT OF SODIUM (SALT) WHEN YOUR SUGGESTED DAILY AMOUNT IS AROUND 2000 MGS. INSTEAD, GET A SLICE OR TWO OF <u>FRESH</u> THIN CRUST CHEESE AND TOMATO PIZZA!

And finally, a big favorite: ice cream. There are some really great lower calorie and low-fat versions on the market. Just to show you the difference, here's a label from Häagen-Dazs Vanilla and Dreyer's Grand Light Vanilla.

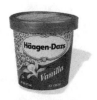
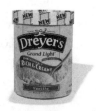

Nutrition Facts

Serving Size 1/2 cup (106g)
Servings Per Container 4

Amount Per Serving

Calories 270	Calories from Fat 160

	% Daily Value*
Total Fat 18g	28%
Saturated Fat 11g	55%
Cholesterol 120mg	40%
Sodium 70mg	3%
Total Carbohydrate 21g	7%
Dietary Fiber 0g	0%
Sugars 21g	
Protein 5g	

Nutrition Facts

Serving Size: 1/2 cup (60g)
Servings Per Container 14

Amount Per Serving

Calories 100	Calories from Fat 30

	% Daily Value*
Total Fat 3.5g	5%
Saturated Fat 2g	10%
Cholesterol 20mg	7%
Sodium 45mg	2%
Total Carbohydrate 15g	5%
Dietary Fiber 0g	0%
Sugars 11g	
Protein 3g	

HÄAGEN-DAZS ICE CREAM

NEARLY TRIPLE THE CALORIES OF DRYER'S LIGHT. AND THOSE FAT AND SATURATED FAT AMOUNTS ARE PAINFULLY HIGH!

DREYER'S LIGHT

A GREAT SNACK THAT FITS OUR 100 CALORIE/LESS THAN 5 GRAMS OF FAT GUIDELINE FOR SNACKS!

A good general rule when you're buying and eating convenience foods like these is to limit your intake of calories, fat, and sodium in *each serving.*

	CALORIES	FAT	SODIUM
1400-CALORIE CATEGORY LIMITS	350	8 gm	400mg
1600-CALORIE CATEGORY LIMITS	400	10 gm	600 mg
2000-CALORIE CATEGORY LIMITS	500	12 gm	800 mg

Now that you're label smart, take it one step further and watch out for these ingredients that we don't recommend for this diet.

FOODS TO AVOID

 High fructose corn syrup

 Hydrogenated oils

 Artificial sweeteners

 Some saturated fats like cottonseed and palm oil

 Fried foods

Here's why you'd be smart to avoid them.

HIGH FRUCTOSE CORN SYRUP

It's everywhere. Drinks, sodas, Popsicles, candy, pancake syrup, fruit-flavored yogurt, pasta sauces, apple juices, and more. Scientific studies have shown that fructose causes weight gain and fat storage because it's metabolized into fat in the liver, rather than absorbed and turned into glucose the way regular sugar is. Solution? Check labels, especially on drinks, and look for products without high fructose corn syrup.

HYDROGENATED OILS

The more hydrogenated oils you have in your diet, the higher your risks are for developing health problems like heart disease and certain cancers. Check the ingredients on nutrition labels: if you see the word hydrogenated, it means trans fatty acids. Stay away!

ARTICIAL SWEETENERS

Aspartame, Equal, NutraSweet, Splenda, Sweet'n Low—ban them all from your diet! They have been targeted as possible culprits in weight gain and obesity. In a recent study at Purdue University, scientists found that rats who ate artificial sweeteners ate three times more calories than the rats who were given real sugar! Why? The scientists think the engineered sweeteners interfere with the body's natural ability to regulate food and calorie intake.

According to the *Journal of the American Medical Association*, a recent study involving 80,000 women over the course of 6 years showed that the more artificial sweetener a woman consumed, the more likely she was to *gain* weight!

The only sweetener we recommend is one called Stevia Plus. You'll most likely find it in health food stores. It's an herb that has been used for hundreds of years in South America. This sweetener is better than the others because it's not artificial and doesn't trigger fat-conserving insulin production. (Insulin, by the way, is a hormone in the pancreas that regulates the level of sugars in the blood.)

SOME SATURATED FATS (COTTONSEED AND PALM OILS)

Cottonseed and palm oils are found in some baked goods and prepared foods. Eating too much of these kinds of fat isn't good for your body because they can clog arteries and make you gain weight.

FRIED FOODS

Fried foods tend to use a lot of oil, which add lots of fat and calories.

Now that you know which foods to avoid, here are the products that we highly recommend for this diet. In fact, they are our top ten favorite store-bought foods—not just because they meet this diet's nutrition standards, but because they taste really good! Promise! You'll find some of them in regular grocery stores, and for others you'll have to go to specialty or health food stores.

PRIA BARS

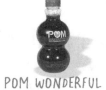

POM WONDERFUL

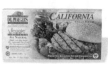

DR. PRAEGER
VEGGIE BURGER

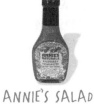

ANNIE'S SALAD
DRESSING

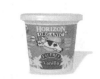

HORIZON ORGANIC
VANILLA YOGURT

HEALTHY CHOICE
SOUPS

FRUIT WATERS

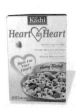

KASHI HEART
TO HEART CEREAL

CLASSICO
SPAGHETTI SAUCE

LEMONAISE
LIGHT

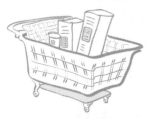

143

All right, now you know how to read labels better and you have some great nutritional foods on your grocery list. A few words of caution (you've probably heard them before): avoid shopping when you're hungry! Your hungry tummy might distract you from making good decisions. If you do find yourself in a grocery store when you're ravenous or needing a little boost, go for the food that your body will be able to use to your best advantage!

TOP FIVE WAYS TO MAKE FOOD WORK FOR YOU

WANT ENERGY? — EAT PROTEINS AND CARBS TOGETHER, LIKE CHEESE AND FRUIT.

WANT TO THINK CLEARLY? — EAT COMPLEX CARBS, LIKE A WHOLE GRAIN ENGLISH MUFFIN OR 8 WHOLE WHEAT CRACKERS.

WANT A STRONG BODY? — DRINK LOW-FAT MILK

WANT TO FEEL FULL? — EAT GARBANZO BEANS, OR FILL UP ON A BOWL OF NON-CREAM VEGETABLE SOUP. LOW-FAT POPCORN WORKS, TOO!

FEEL A COLD COMING ON? — BOOST YOUR CITRUS INTAKE! ORANGES, STRAWBERRIES, AND THE NUMBER ONE VITAMIN C KING OF FRUITS—KIWI!

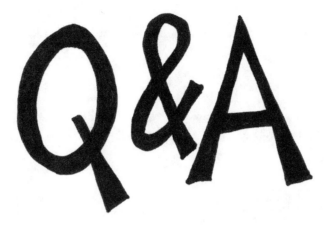

Q&A

IS THERE REALLY A BIG DIFFERENCE BETWEEN ORGANIC AND REGULAR FOODS? ORGANIC IS MORE EXPENSIVE.

Organic means foods that have been produced without using pesticides, chemicals, or extra hormones. That's good. It is more expensive, but worth it—especially with dairy products. But don't worry if you can't afford organic products; it's not the end of the world, just be sure to wash your fruits and vegetables well.

WHAT DO THE LABELS "LIGHT," "LOW-FAT," AND "REDUCED CALORIES" MEAN?

 "Light" means the product has either $1/3$ fewer calories or half the fat of the original food. If it says "light sodium," that means the salt content has been reduced by half.

"Low-fat" means 3 grams of fat or less per serving.

 "Reduced calories" means 25 percent fewer calories than the original food.

ARE FROZEN FOODS AND CANNED FOODS OKAY TO EAT?

Fresh is always best, but actually frozen isn't all that bad. Here's why. Frozen foods are harvested then immediately frozen on the spot at packaging plants, so lots of nutrients stay in. As for canned foods, try eating them only when there's no other choice. Usually canned foods have lots of preservatives and salt.

I'VE HEARD THAT YOU'RE NOT SUPPOSED TO EAT CANNED TUNA.

There have been reports that tuna fish has high levels of mercury, a mineral you don't want a lot of in your system because it makes it harder for your kidneys and liver to work properly, plus it can affect concentration and memory. Canned tuna is okay to eat once or twice a week. Buying "chunk light" instead of albacore cuts back the mercury levels.

I FEEL STUPID, BUT WHEN I READ A LABEL AND IT SAYS STUFF LIKE "CHOLESTEROL 30 MGS," I HAVE NO IDEA WHAT THAT MEANS. ACTUALLY, THE WHOLE LABEL CONFUSES ME!

Don't feel stupid, *very* few people can figure that stuff out. Let's clarify. Here's the approximate amount of what everybody needs when it comes to fiber, cholesterol, and sodium, as well as protein, carbohydrates, and fats.

 Fiber = about 25 grams per day

 Cholesterol = no more than 300 mgs per day

 Sodium = no more than 2000 mgs per day

(The daily suggested amounts of protein, carbohydrates, and fat vary per calorie category.)

	1400	1600	2000
PROTEIN	105 g	120 g	150 g
CARBOHYDRATES	175 g	200 g	250 g
FAT	31 g	35 g	44 g

HOW DO I FIND OUT HOW MUCH SUGAR IS IN A PRODUCT? ALL THEY LIST IS GRAMS. AND HOW MUCH SUGAR SHOULD BE IN MY DIET?

Great questions. Look at the nutrition label and find out how many grams of sugar are in a serving. Dividing that number by 4 will give you the amount in teaspoons. A 12-ounce can of soda has about 40 grams of sugar. That's a whopping 10 teaspoons!

The USDA recommends limiting sugar in your diet to 6 to 10 percent of your daily calorie amount. One teaspoon of sugar equals 16 calories. So here are your suggested daily limits and how much sugar is in certain foods.

1400 calories a day	6 to 9 teaspoons a day
1600 calories a day	6 to 10 teaspoons a day
2000 calories a day	8 to 12 teaspoons a day

1 doughnut	4 teaspoons
1 slice cheesecake	11 teaspoons
1 cookie	3 teaspoons
1 cup sweetened cereal	3 teaspoons

FOOD FOR THOUGHT: DESSERTS IS STRESSED SPELLED BACKWARD!

SEVEN | YOU GOT SERVED...

Chances are you're getting *huge* servings of food, whether you're at a restaurant, a deli, the mall, or McDonald's. Even at most vending machines, you're being sold big gobs of poor nutrition. Did you know that marketers have been trying to manipulate you into craving their products ever since you were a kid?

You've been bombarded by TV ads that show bowls and plates overflowing with food. You've seen countless commercials where kids are guzzling giant-size sodas, eating big bags of candy, digging into huge ice cream sundaes—looking as happy as can be. Most movie theaters sell large popcorn buckets that actually hold the equivalent of thirty normal servings!

And soft drink sizes have been super-sized from 4½ ounces to 18 ounces per serving. Pizzas are often sold two for one. In grocery stores, certain manufacturers pay big bucks to place their heavily advertised products on store shelves at eye level for children, so that they will see these foods and beg their parents to buy them.

Advertisers don't care about your nutrition. They just want to sell products, selling you and your health out in the process. Don't let these clever marketers fool you! You can do better! Don't justify bad food choices and feel forced to eat what's available. Take the lead. Cut your portions in half. Make smart choices.

RESTAURANT GUIDELINES

1. Ask for sauces and salad dressings on the side; or make your own by mixing 1 teaspoon of the restaurant's dressing with any variety of vinegar.

2. Use condiments like salsa and mustard instead of mayonnaise and oil.

3. Use non- or low-fat milk.

4. Order baked or grilled lean meats instead of fried or fatty ones.

5. Order two appetizers as your main meal.

6. Ask for half portions.

7. Order a sandwich with lean meats, chicken, turkey, tuna (made with low-fat mayonnaise), lean ham, or roast beef. Eat it open faced, with the meat on top of a single slice of bread.

8. Remove the bread basket from the table.

9. Order soups that aren't cream-based.

10. Order pasta with marinara (tomato sauce).

11. Ask for the kid-size portion.

12. Never have seconds at buffet-style restaurants.

13. Have fruit for dessert.

14. Avoid ordering foods that are breaded, deep-fried, coated, or creamy (like Alfredo sauce on pasta), which contain a lot of fat. In general, restaurant meals are full of fat because cooking with fat is an easy way to make food taste good.

15. Don't think you have to finish what's on your plate because you paid for it. Ask for a doggy bag and make it another meal the next day.

Here's a general breakdown of what to eat and what to avoid at specialty food vendors and restaurants.

DELIS

 EAT THIS NOT THAT

EAT THIS	NOT THAT
SLICED CHICKEN	CHICKEN SALAD WITH MAYONNAISE
WHOLE GRAIN BREAD OR BAGEL	CROISSANTS
½ BAKED HAM SANDWICH	CORNED BEEF, BOLOGNA, OR PASTRAMI
½ ROASTED TURKEY SANDWICH	SANDWICHES
NON-CREAM-BASED SOUP	POTATO SOUP

SALAD BAR

 EAT THIS NOT THAT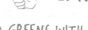

EAT THIS	NOT THAT
MIXED GREENS WITH LOW-FAT DRESSING	HIGH-FAT DRESSINGS LIKE BLUE CHEESE, RANCH, AND THOUSAND ISLAND
CHICKPEAS OR ANY BEANS	PASTA SALAD
FRESH VEGETABLES	MARINATED VEGETABLES

EAT THIS	NOT THAT
EGG WHITES	WHOLE EGGS
TURKEY BITS	BACON BITS
NUTS OR SEEDS	CROUTONS
FETA, GOAT, OR MOZZARELLA CHEESE	CHEDDAR CHEESE

MEXICAN FOOD

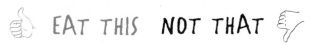

EAT THIS   NOT THAT

EAT THIS	NOT THAT
SALSA	SALAD DRESSING
LOW-FAT SOUR CREAM	REGULAR SOUR CREAM
FAJITAS	CHIMICHANGAS
BURRITO WITH NO CHEESE OR LOW-FAT CHEESE	REGULAR BURRITO
SOFT CHICKEN TACOS	CRISPY TACOS

CHINESE FOOD

 EAT THIS   NOT THAT

EAT THIS	NOT THAT
HOT AND SPICY ANYTHING	DEEP-FRIED ANYTHING
STEAMED/SAUTÉED SHRIMP OR CHICKEN	BREADED SHRIMP, CHICKEN, OR PORK
WONTON SOUP	EGG DROP SOUP
STIR-FRY WITH LIGHT OIL	FRIED CRISPY NOODLES
FORTUNE COOKIE	ALMOND COOKIE

JAPANESE FOOD

 EAT THIS   NOT THAT

EAT THIS	NOT THAT
MISO SOUP	SUKIYAKI (IF MADE WITH FATTY MEAT)
SASHIMI	TEMPURA (BATTER-FRIED)
SUSHI	DYNAMOS (CREAM-BASED COOKED FISH DISH)
CHICKEN TERIYAKI	BEEF TERIYAKI

MALL FOOD

 EAT THIS   NOT THAT

EAT THIS	NOT THAT
BAKED POTATO WITH SALSA	BAKED POTATO WITH CHEESE OR SOUR CREAM
THIN-CRUST PIZZA WITH LIGHT CHEESE	THICK-CRUST PIZZA WITH PEPPERONI
SMALL, LOW-FAT BLUEBERRY MUFFIN	LARGE CHOCOLATE MUFFIN
FISH TACOS (UNBREADED FILLING WITH SOFT TORTILLA)	BREADED FISH TACOS (WITH FRIED SHELL)

FAST FOOD

(EAT ONLY WHEN IN A JAM, AND NEVER MORE THAN ONCE A WEEK.)

 EAT THIS   NOT THAT

EAT THIS	NOT THAT
VEGGIE BURGER ON HALF A BUN	DOUBLE ANYTHING
SMALL BEAN BURRITO	BEAN, CHEESE, AND RICE BURRITO
SALAD WITH NONFAT DRESSING	SALADS WITH CRISPY NOODLES OR CHEESE DRESSING
CHICKEN BREAST SANDWICH ON HALF A BUN	BREADED CHICKEN SANDWICH

NOTE: EATING FAST FOOD MORE THAN TWICE A WEEK INCREASES YOUR CHANCE OF BECOMING OBESE BY 50 PERCENT!!!

FROZEN FOODS

 EAT THIS   NOT THAT

BRANDS LIKE AMY'S, CASCADIAN FARMS, CEDARLANE NATURE FOODS, AND HEALTHY CHOICE

BRANDS WITH LABELS THAT SHOW LOTS OF FAT AND/OR SODIUM (SALT)

SCHOOL CAFETERIA

 EAT THIS   NOT THAT

YOUR OWN PACKED LUNCH

MACARONI AND CHEESE, DEEP-FRIED FOODS

STEAMED VEGETABLES

VEGETABLES WITH CREAM SAUCE

FRESH FRUIT

HIGH-SUGAR FRUIT CUPS

UNBREADED FISH OR CHICKEN (REMOVE BREADING YOURSELF.)

BREADED CHICKEN OR FISH

*TRY TO CHOOSE HIGH-DENSITY NUTRITIOUS FOODS LIKE A LOW-FAT STRING CHEESE OR AN APPLE INSTEAD OF EMPTY CALORIE ITEMS LIKE COLAS AND HIGH SUGAR FOODS. PUT SNACKS IN BAGGIES TO KEEP YOUR PORTION SIZES RIGHT, AND KEEP THEM IN YOUR BACKPACK, CAR, OR SCHOOL LOCKER IN CASE YOU GET HUNGRY AND NEED TO REACH FOR THE CLOSEST THING TO EAT.

VENDING MACHINES

Vending machines might be convenient (fast food when you're in a hurry), but as far as nutrition goes, most of them score a big fat F. Why? Vendors need to put products in their machines that will sell and last a long time, which means they contain lots of unhealthy preservatives and chemicals.

But let's say you forgot your lunch. You're starving and this is the only option left. If you absolutely, positively, really and truly can't find anything else to eat, talk to yourself in front of the vending machine!

As for vending machine beverages, be careful of sodas and juice drinks with high fructose corn syrup—not a good form of sugar. (You'll learn more about that later in this chapter.) Go for water and *forget sodas*, diet or regular! If you only do one thing after you've read this book, do this: **Stop drinking sodas, especially diet sodas!** All the regular sodas offer you is sugar (up to 12 teaspoons in one can, which is several teaspoons more than your daily allowance!) and empty calories. Diet sodas are full of artificial

CHEETOS? HMM...WHERE'S THE CHEESE? IT'S ALL ARTIFICIAL, HIGH FAT, HIGH CALORIES. NO!

PRETZELS, A CARB SNACK FOR ENERGY...YES!

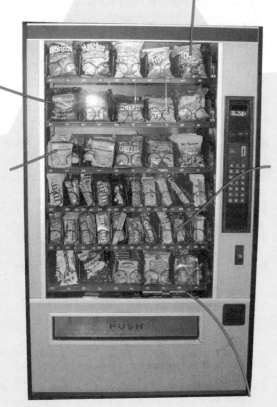

TOP RAMEN, HMM... HIGH IN SALT, BUT IT'S ACTUALLY A GOOD MINI MEAL IF YOU'RE IN A PINCH.

THIS HONEY AND OAT GRANOLA BAR LOOKS HEALTHY...AND IT IS! GOOD CHOICE. YES!

CANDY BARS, COOKIES, AND DOUGHNUTS. REALLY BAD CHOICES. TOO MUCH SUGAR, FAT, AND CALORIES.

sweeteners, colors, and flavors—nothing natural. Plus, sodas can mess up your body! Here's what can happen if you drink lots of soda (and, for that matter, juice drinks with high fructose sugar).

1. **YOUR BONES CAN BECOME WEAKER.** Scientists have found that active girls who drink carbonated beverages, especially colas, are *five times* more likely to have bone fractures! According to the Harvard School of Public Health, certain ingredients in colas can hinder bone development. Considering the fact that 90 percent of your bone mass is built by the age of seventeen, this is prime time to treat your bones right!

2. **YOU'RE AT RISK FOR DEVELOPING TYPE 2 DIABETES.** A study published in the *Journal of the American Medical Association* found that women who regularly drink sugar-sweetened sodas gained more weight and had a greater risk of developing type 2 diabetes than those who didn't or hardly ever drank high-sugar drinks.

3. **YOU MIGHT GET CELLULITE.** Cellulite is actually normal fat. It looks bumpy because it's pushing through the connective tissues beneath your skin. The thickness of your skin, your age, and genetics all help determine whether you'll develop cellulite, and how much. But eating less saturated fat (fatty meats and fried

foods), drinking more water, and avoiding diet sodas might reduce cellulite.

4. **THE CAFFEINE CAN MAKE YOU FIDGETY AND ANXIOUS.**

Too much caffeine can give you the jitters and even lead to insomnia.

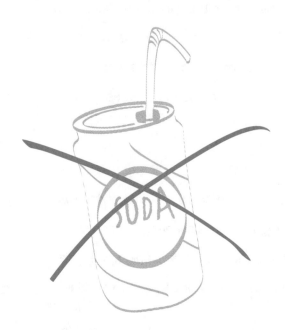

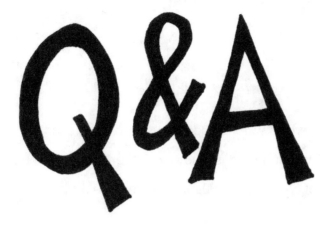

Q&A

SHOULD I DRINK GATORADE OR SIMILAR DRINKS?

Probably not, unless you're an athlete, and even then there are better sports drinks like Recharge that have less fructose sugars and no additives. Gatorade actually contains some trans fats, as well as artificial flavors and dye. Reach for more natural drinks like Mountain Spring and flavored waters.

WHAT ABOUT ALCOHOL? DOES IT MATTER IF I HAVE A BEER OR A DRINK AT PARTIES?

Alcoholic drinks are bad for you for a number of reasons, especially in terms of nutrition. They contain calories that have no nutritional value and will turn to fat very quickly. Drinking will also distract you from making good food decisions. So no alcohol on this diet.

NO SODAS, NO HIGH FRUCTOSE CORN SYRUP DRINKS, NO ALCOHOL . . . WHAT DO I DRINK?

Drink decaf iced tea with no sugar or use the sweetener stevia. The Fruit Waters by Glacéau brand is also good. We like the Calistoga flavored waters, and of course our exclusive Pom Tea (see recipe in chapter 5).

I GET THESE INSANE CRAVINGS FOR THINGS LIKE LASAGNA OR PASTA WITH ALFREDO SAUCE. WHAT SHOULD I DO?

You don't have to deny yourself. Just don't eat huge portions. If you're going to indulge, order a child-size portion or split the meal with someone.

Now, just in case fast food is your only option, here's a reference list to show you the amount of calories, fat, carbohydrates, and protein you'll find in foods served at some of the most popular restaurant chains. Note that we're only listing the foods that can even remotely be considered okay for you to eat. Remember, we don't recommend fast food more than once a week. Always ask to have the following foods taken off your dish: mayonnaise, cheese, special sauces, dressing, croutons, butter, and sour cream.

MCDONALD'S

	CALORIES	FAT	CARBS	PROTEIN
CHICKEN MCGRILL	300	6g	37g	25g
CAESAR SALAD W/ GRILLED CHICKEN (W/O DRESSING)	210	7g	11g	26g
FRUIT 'N YOGURT PARFAIT (W/O GRANOLA)	280	4g	53g	8g
SNACK-SIZE FRUIT 'N YOGURT PARFAIT	160	2g	30g	4g
W/O GRANOLA	130	2g	25g	4g

JACK IN THE BOX

	CALORIES	FAT	CARBS	PROTEIN
CHICKEN FAJITA PITA	330	11g	35g	24g
TACO	170	9g	15g	6g

BURGER KING

	CALORIES	FAT	CARBS	PROTEIN
CHICKEN WHOPPER	420	9g	47g	38g
BK VEGGIE BURGER	310	7g	46g	15g
CHICKEN CAESAR	160	6g	5g	25g

CARL'S JR.

	CALORIES	FAT	CARBS	PROTEIN
HAMBURGER	280	9g	36g	14g
CHARBROILED BBQ CHICKEN SANDWICH	290	3.5g	41g	25g
CHARBROILED CHICKEN SALAD-TO-GO	200	7g	12g	25g
GARDEN SALAD-TO-GO	50	2.5g	4g	3g
ENGLISH MUFFIN	210	9g	28g	5g

PIZZA HUT

1 THIN 'N CRISPY PIZZA SLICE = 1 SERVING

	CALORIES	FAT	CARBS	PROTEIN
CHEESE	200	9g	22g	10g
HAM	170	7g	21g	9g
VEGGIE LOVER'S	190	7g	24g	8g
SPAGHETTI WITH MARINARA	490	6g	91g	18g

TACO BELL

	CALORIES	FAT	CARBS	PROTEIN
SOFT BEEF TACO	210	10g	21g	11g
SOFT CHICKEN TACO	190	6g	19g	14g
TOSTADA	250	10g	29g	11g

SUBWAY

SUBWAY SANDWICHES INCLUDING ITALIAN OR WHEAT BREAD, LETTUCE, TOMATOES, ONIONS, GREEN PEPPER, OLIVES, AND PICKLES

	CALORIES	FAT	CARBS	PROTEIN
6" HAM	290	5g	46g	18g
6" ROASTED TURKEY	290	5g	45g	19g
6" CHICKEN BREAST	320	5g	47g	23g
6" VEGGIE DELITE	230	3g	44g	9g
HAM ON DELI ROUND BREAD	210	4g	35g	11g
ROAST BEEF ON DELI ROUND BREAD	220	4.5g	35g	13g
TURKEY BREAST ON DELI ROUND BREAD	220	3.5g	36g	13g
6" CHICKEN TERIYAKI	380	5g	59g	26g

WENDY'S

	CALORIES	FAT	CARBS	PROTEIN
JR. HAMBURGER	270	9g	14g	34g
GRILLED CHICKEN SANDWICH	300	7g	36g	24g
MANDARIN CHICKEN SALAD	348	1.5g	17g	20g
SPRING MIX SALAD	180	11g	12g	11g
PLAIN BAKED POTATO	310	0g	72g	7g

CHICK-FIL-A

	CALORIES	FAT	CARBS	PROTEIN
CHAR-GRILLED CHICKEN COOL WRAP	380	6g	54g	29g
CHAR-GRILLED CHICKEN GARDEN SALAD	180	6g	9g	22g
CHAR-GRILLED CHICKEN SANDWICH	250	3g	28g	26g

IF YOU WISH TO GROW THINNER, DIMINISH YOUR DINNER.

—H. S. LEIGH

MY BOYFRIEND DUMPED ME, AND I CAN'T STOP EATING *EIGHT*

I WOULD FINALLY BE ALONE AND THEN EAT AN
ENTIRE BAG OF CHIPS PLUS A FULL CONTAINER OF
ONION DIP. IT MADE ME FEEL BETTER AT FIRST. THEN
I'D FEEL HORRIBLE AFTER.

—ANONYMOUS

This is how one of the girls in our survey reacted when her boyfriend broke

up with her to date one of her friends. She felt lost, out of control, and dev-

astated. Eating made her feel good for a minute, then it made her feel hor-

rible and ashamed. She was caught in a vicious cycle.

169

It's not just boyfriend trouble that can mess with your eating habits; it can be lots of different things. You might feel rejected by a friend or scared about growing up. You might have family issues or school troubles. Perhaps you're bored, lonely, or even depressed. These serious emotions can hit hard and really hurt.

If no one has taught you how to deal with them or if you're feeling these complex emotions for the first time, you might not know what to do. If you "stuff" your feelings down, they'll eventually come out, usually in unhealthy ways—like unexplained outbursts of anger, irritability, overeating, or even starving yourself.

People who've experienced this will tell you the best way to handle emotional damage is to get help and be very, very aware of what's happening to you. Be kind to yourself, and pay attention to what you're feeling. Write down what's going on inside, talk to people, get the emotions out. Go for a walk or run, or punch something like a pillow or punching bag. Remember, it's okay to have negative feelings or thoughts, but it's what you do with them that counts.

Know that no matter how hard you're crying or how miserable you feel, the worst part—that intense feeling of despair—will generally last about 20 minutes, and then give way to a new feeling. You will get through it whether you want to or not, so try to hang in there and take comfort in that. The pain will come and go, and at moments you'll feel like the whole world has just crashed around you and left you spinning.

A lot of people turn to food when they're sad or depressed because eating offers instant gratification. But food only offers a quick fix; eating when you're depressed is kind of like putting a Band-Aid on a broken arm. You're not really dealing with the issues. Stuffing food into your body or starving it isn't going to fix the real problems.

Try to deal with the issues that are bugging you. If you can, see a professional like a therapist. If money is an issue, contact your local United Way and ask for counseling help. They can try to get you low-cost or free therapy. Search out self-help books in bookstores, go online to get information, and maybe find a hotline that you can call for help.

But when it comes to food, be very honest with yourself. As you reach for that snack, ask yourself "Am I really hungry?" The answer to that question is trickier than it may seem. Surprisingly, most people eat when they're *not* really hungry. They eat when they're upset or bored, or because something smells good, or simply because everyone else is eating.

Test this theory on yourself. Notice *when* you eat and *why*. Are you really hungry, or is something apart from hunger prompting you to eat? Identify your "food triggers" and keep track of them in your diet journal. It could be seeing an ad, or automatically reaching for an after-school snack, or munching while you're on the Internet. You should be aware of these triggers—whatever they are—and learn to outsmart them!

So before you turn to food, always ask yourself, "Am I really hungry? Or am I bored or sad or depressed?" If the answer is yes to the second question, try facing those emotions directly.

EAT WHEN YOU'RE HUNGRY. WHEN YOU'RE NOT, STOP.

DID YOU KNOW THERE ARE TWO KINDS OF HUNGER?

TRUE HUNGER

The first sign of true hunger is a little twinge or cramp in your stomach, maybe some gurgling. This could mean your stomach is empty and it's time to eat. If you ignore this feeling for too long, you risk bingeing and wanting to eat everything in sight!

EMOTIONAL HUNGER

One of the best ways of dealing with emotional hunger is understanding it. Emotional hunger is a feeling deep down inside that somehow food is going to make you feel better and solve internal problems like depression, loneliness, or stress. We're fans of the author Geneen Roth, who knows a lot about emotional eating. Here's an excerpt from her website www.geneenroth.com.

So many emotional eaters have a sense of never getting enough. They approach life from an inner sense of poverty, and no amount of food, sex, clothes, or money will satisfy them. I ask them to question the notion of being forever deprived, to recognize that it is in their minds, though probably based on a real experience of having felt deprived in the past. As a child, I couldn't get enough of my mother's love. But I was not in control of my mother. As an adult, I was in control of how much food I ate, so I ate more to make up for not having had enough of something vital in my past: in this case, love. I felt deprived and poverty-stricken when it came to love, and that became part of my motivation for eating compulsively. For the first twenty-five years of my life, I had a constant feeling that I could not get enough. Realizing that I could get enough food—and still lose weight—was a major turning point. If you want to lose weight, you can do it by eating only when you're hungry and stopping when you've had enough. But this thought is frightening to most people, because it means taking responsibility and trusting yourself.

So if you're eating for the wrong reasons, here are ways to out-smart tricky cravings. Our favorite one is called:

DELAY . . . THEN DECIDE

Here's an example of "Delay . . . then decide:" Let's say you're ravenous for McDonald's food. You're about to hit the drive-through. Your stomach is saying, "Man, I can't wait for that cheeseburger!" Your brain is saying, "Man, I shouldn't have those calories, that fat, those fries!"

THIS IS THE TIME TO DELAY! As in drive away. Yup, just drive away and decide later. You'll be surprised to find that, after just a few minutes, you'll be able to make a better decision because you won't be acting on impulse. Imagine how good you'll feel afterward about making a healthy decision and not giving in to instant gratification.

Other ways to delay:

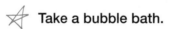 **Take a bubble bath.**

Read a fitness/health magazine.

Make a cup of tea.

Dance or sing to your favorite music.

Give yourself a manicure or pedicure.

Write a poem, or write in a journal.

 Do sit-ups.

 Meditate.

 Go for a walk.

If you've tried *all* of this and are still having a monster craving . . . well, go ahead and have a piece of the dang thing, but make it small. And make it the exception, not the rule.

TOP SIX DIET TRAPS

1. SOCIAL EVENTS

You're out to dinner or at an event with your friends and they're all eating lots of food, or you're at a party with a big buffet. You're tempted to go wild and eat whatever is in sight. Stick to your guns, girl! Do what's right for *your* nutritional needs, and don't cave in to peer pressure.

2. YOU'RE HUNGRY

You're depriving yourself or simply not getting enough to eat, and you get ravenously hungry. It's hard for you to control yourself when powerful

175

forces like that come into play. Try not to let your hunger get to that point. On this diet—and for the rest of your life—you should be fueling your body throughout the day.

3. YOU'RE TIRED, DISTRACTED, OR BORED

You're grabbing whatever food is conveniently in reach because you don't feel like taking the time to cook or shop for more healthful food, or you tell yourself you've got nothing better to do. Ask yourself if you're *really* hungry. If not, try the delay tactics we suggested. And avoid eating while watching TV, driving, reading, talking on the phone, or sitting in bed—you will be sidetracked and end up eating more food than you need. Make the Zen Mix from chapter 5 or engage in a nonfood activity.

4. YOU DON'T HAVE A PLAN

Each morning, or at the beginning of each week, determine what you will be eating, and when. People who have a plan lose more weight than people who don't.

5. YOUR BODY IS GIVING YOU MIXED SIGNALS

Did you know that your body can give you mixed signals? Sometimes you think you're hungry when you're really thirsty! Give yourself a dehydration test. When you pinch the skin on your elbow, does it spring back into place? If not, you may be dehydrated. Dehydration often makes you tired; your body might mistake this lack of energy for hunger. Try drinking water first.

6. YOU'RE UNAWARE OF FOOD "TRIGGERS"

Ah, the sweet smell of fresh baked pie. Suddenly you're ready to chow down. Wait, you've been triggered! Do you really want to feed your body all of that sugar and fat? Here are some ways to slow down and keep powerful triggers at bay.

- Localize your eating: sit—don't stand!—at the same place when you eat.

- Use a smaller plate.

- Put small bites on your fork or spoon, or use smaller utensils—like a cocktail fork or baby spoon.

- Put your utensils down after each bite, and consciously take time to savor and chew your food.

- Don't ever "clean your plate" just for the sake of it. You are not a dishwasher! Eat until you are full, and then stop.

- Don't eat while driving. You can't really pay attention and enjoy your food. Plus your risk of getting into an accident goes way up.

TEMPTATION IS POWERFUL. YOU'RE MORE POWERFUL.

Some of the savvy girls in our surveys came up with their own ways to handle temptation. One girl says she broke the "clean your plate" habit by pouring water on the food that was leftover on her plate, then adding salt, pepper, and sugar. Suddenly, the food no longer had any power over her.

Another girl said she chewed each bite far more slowly than she normally would. This helped her to realize when she was full.

Another young woman lives by this mantra: "If you don't like the taste, spit it out." She won't waste calories on foods she doesn't love.

But don't beat yourself up if you occasionally succumb to temptation. A normal, healthy diet doesn't require eating exactly the right mix of calories and nutrition *all the time*. Some days you'll get it right, and others you won't. That's normal! The goal is to have more good days than bad.

If you don't eat that well for a day or so, get back on track and remember: **Your next meal is more important than your last one.** Enjoy the food you eat. Trust yourself to make good decisions, in all aspects of your life!

Having said all that, we understand that you'll have those moments when nothing will help—none of our information, no motivational sayings, nothing—and you're going to turn to sweets for companionship. We get that. We've all been there. In that case, try one of these sweet treats below (yes, they do count as part of your daily calories).

BEST "100 CALORIE" FUN TREATS!

1 Tootsie Roll

1 Peppermint Pattie

1 Nerd Rope

20 Gummi Bears

4 red licorice vines

4 big marshmallows

1 cup hot chocolate with low-sugar mix

1 cup decaf cappuccino with low-fat milk

4 Hershey's Chocolate Kisses

Low-fat Kozy Shack Pudding

1 frozen soft pretzel

A big handful of Pirate's Booty snacks

10 Kashi TLC crackers

THERE ARE 3 BILLION WOMEN WHO DON'T LOOK LIKE SUPERMODELS AND ONLY 8 WHO DO. LOVE YOUR BODY.

—EXCERPTED FROM AN AD BY THE BODY SHOP

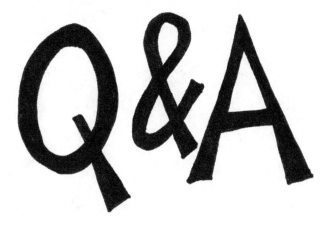

WHAT'S THE PRIMARY CAUSE OF WEIGHT GAIN?

It's emotional eating—like when you're bored or lonely or stressed. Many girls eat when they've just come home from school, or while they're on the Internet or watching TV. You have to become really aware of these triggers and understand them. Sure, it's easy to grab that bag of chips or the carton of ice cream. But stop! Eat an apple or another snack instead. Don't put junk into your body just because it's easy.

ISN'T THE EASIEST WAY TO LOSE WEIGHT TO STARVE MYSELF?

No. Here's why. While you think you're dieting, you're body thinks you're starving and goes into overdrive to conserve everything you do eat. Your metabolism (the speed at which your body burns off calories) slows down and your system is malnourished. Feeding your true hunger keeps your metabolism where it should be, and that helps you burn calories.

BUT WHAT IF I JUST DON'T LIKE THE TASTE OF LOW-SUGAR OR LOW-FAT FOODS? IT'S SO MUCH MORE SATISFYING TO EAT CANDY BARS!

Sure, it may be instantly gratifying to eat junk food *while you're eating it*— but try to imagine how you'll feel afterward: sluggish, unmotivated, and guilty. If your taste buds are used to high-sugar, high-carb foods, it may take a while to "reprogram" them and your eating habits. You can do this by getting used to the low-sugar, low-fat foods. There are fabulous healthful food products on the market that taste great without the junk!

WHY DO I CRAVE CRUNCHY FOODS?

There's such a thing as "mouth feel" which is the way food actually feels in your mouth. It's the texture of food. Your body craves a variety of food textures—like soft, crunchy, smooth, cold, warm, and crispy. Look for low-fat, low-calorie snacks like carrots, rice cakes, or a bowl of soup to satisfy these cravings.

HOW SHOULD I HANDLE THE OVERWHELMING URGE I GET TO EAT SOMETIMES?

If you are truly hungry, then eat something! If not, try all of the tricks we've listed above—and remember, you *will* get a chance to eat again. Relax, your next meal is right around the corner.

I THINK I CAN, I THINK I CAN!

NINE

IF IT WERE EASY TO BE IN GREAT
SHAPE AND LOOK FABULOUS,
EVERYONE WOULD BE.

—OVERHEARD AT A GYM

How true is that? Also true is this mantra: "you gotta move it to lose it!"

There, that says it all, end of chapter! Well, not really. But exercise is

extremely important to your diet and your health. With exercise, you will be able to lose weight more efficiently and effectively. If you're trying to shed pounds, you need to get up out of that chair. If you're not trying to shed pounds, but don't play sports or get out much, you'll also benefit from exercise.

There's no way to sugar-coat it. It might be hard to motivate yourself, at first. You'll need willpower and determination. If you're a couch potato, becoming physically active won't happen overnight. You'll have to stick with an exercise plan until it becomes a part of you—and you see the benefits and start feeling empowered. Some people never reach that point; they give up after a few workouts. But many people find their way to a healthier, more active lifestyle.

Here's an inspiring story about one girl who made the transition. She was very overweight, over 350 pounds. It was tough for her to exercise, and she didn't have good eating habits. She also needed a job. When she finally got one, it was—of all places—at a gym! The owner needed a receptionist, and he liked this girl's warm personality. (He was one of the few people who looked past her appearance.)

It was uncomfortable for her at first, being around people who were so much more fit. But after a few weeks, one day she just got up from her desk and walked to the back of a class that the owner was teaching. She stood there. People stared. The music started. The other people started exercising. And she did too, although all she could do was lift her legs a little bit. But she kept at it for the duration of the session. Then, with tears in her eyes and to the applause of the entire class—she went back to her desk.

It was a breakthrough moment. She had finally decided to do something about her body and her health, and it made all the difference in the world. She eventually ended up losing a lot of weight. Although she never became really thin (which probably wouldn't have been natural for her), she became much fitter and healthier—and, no doubt, more confident.

We cannot stress enough how important exercise is to a healthy lifestyle, especially if you want to lose weight. We could give you countless statistics on the benefits of working out that would make your eyes glaze over. But our favorite benefit, the one that will really help motivate you, is this: Exercise can change your brain chemistry! When you get your heartrate going with serious exercise, your body releases endorphins, which are natural pain-relieving hormones that make you feel "naturally high." You'll feel calmer, less anxious, and more confident after you've worked out.

Among doctors and fitness experts, the general consensus is that you should work out at least three times a week for 20 to 40 minutes. That means playing sports or exercising vigorously enough to break a sweat and get your heart pumping. Choose exercise activities that are fun for you, so you'll find it easier to stick to your routine.

Strength training is an important part of a workout, not only for muscle health, but for boosting your metabolism—and self-esteem! Keep in mind we're not talking about becoming body builders, those kinds of workouts are too intense for your growing body. We'll show you how to incorporate weights into your work-out routine, so that you can build some muscle tone and enhance your dieting efforts.

But first, just as we suggested that you check with your doctor before starting a new diet, we suggest that you get a health check-up before starting a new exercise program.

WORKING OUT REGULARLY WILL....

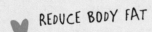 REDUCE BODY FAT

INCREASE YOUR ENERGY LEVEL

MAKE YOUR COMPLEXION GLOW

RELEASE "ENDORPHINS," WHICH WILL GIVE YOU A "NATURAL HIGH"

MAKE YOUR BODY MORE IMMUNE TO GERMS AND ILLNESSES

MAKE YOUR BRAIN WORK BETTER

MAKE YOUR CLOTHES FIT BETTER

188

The following mini-training program was developed exclusively for this book by Tina Angelotti, a former gymnast and fitness coach to teenagers, who is now a certified and accredited Los Angeles trainer. She runs a program at the wildly popular Krav Maga Self-Defense Center.

Your workout will consist of three main types of exercise:

1. CARDIOVASCULAR ("cardio" for short): Get your heart pumping for about 20 minutes per workout.

2. STRENGTH Work the muscles of your entire body, especially your "core," meaning the muscles and abs (abdominal muscles) around your spine, for about 10 minutes per workout.

3. FLEXIBILITY Stretch your muscles for about 10 minutes per workout.

Follow this routine 3 to 5 times a week for about 40 minutes per session.

CARDIO: MAKE YOUR HEART STRONGER!

Cardiovascular respiratory fitness is the kind of exercise that gets your heart beating at a faster than normal rate and speeds up your breathing.

As your heart pumps blood more quickly and forcefully to all your working muscles, your body must use up energy to keep going. Since calories are a form of energy (as we discussed in chapter 3), the more energy you use to exercise, the more calories you burn!

The good news is that cardio exercise will get easier with practice, and yet you'll still be burning up the same number of calories. So keep going!

There is such a thing as a plateau, however. You know you've reached it when you've been doing the same exercise and eating right, but can't seem to lose weight. This is a good time to kick your fitness plan into higher gear or try some new workout to give your body the message that it's time to start burning calories again.

But if you're just starting an exercise program (and your doctor has approved it), start out easy, then gradually work your way up to doing cardio training 3 to 5 times per week, for anywhere between 20 to 40 minutes per session. Here's a good way to do this.

For beginners, start with 60 seconds of slow jogging, followed by 60 seconds of walking, and continue alternating jogging and walking for a total of 20 minutes. (If the jogging part is too tough, try just walking briskly.) Gradually work up to doing this same workout for a total of 30 minutes. To make it a little more challenging, increase your jogging to 90-second intervals instead of 60-second ones.

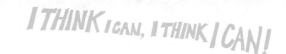

- ✦ If you're a more advanced exerciser, try alternating 5 minutes of jogging with 1 minute of walking for a total of 20 minutes. Gradually work your way up to a brisk jog for the full 20 minutes.

- ✦ If you enjoy competition, try timing how long it takes you to run or jog a mile, then try to beat your time the following week. Exercising with a friend can also motivate you to push yourself harder.

(If you don't like jogging, try some other type of cardio exercise for 20 minutes—like using the treadmill, elliptical, or stairstepper machines. As you get more advanced, work up to 40 minutes.)

STRENGTH: MAKE YOUR MUSCLES STRONGER!

Basic strength training (again, we're not talking body building here!) will help increase your metabolism; your body will burn calories much more efficiently with strong muscles. This type of exercise will also stabilize your joints and strengthen your tendons, which is important for preventing common injuries when you're exercising or leading an active life.

But the *best* benefit of strength training is increased athletic performance. Whatever you do, whatever sport you play—or if you dance—you'll do it better and it will seem easier if you've got stronger muscles. You'll jump higher, run faster, move with more agility, and lift things with more ease!

Strength training starts with "core" training. Your core is the part of your body where all of your movement originates—that is, all of the muscles around your spine. Not just the abdominals muscles, but also the muscles that lie beneath the six-pack!

CORE TRAINING EXERCISES

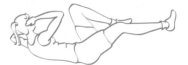

1. THE BICYCLE: Lie flat on your back, knees bent, hands holding your head at the sides behind the ears. Lift your head and slowly start bringing your knees, one at a time, to the opposite elbow.

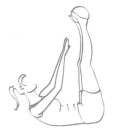
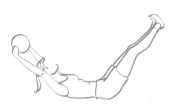

2. V-UP: While on your back, hold a ball or pillow between your hands, pass it to your feet, lower feet with ball or pillow between them, then pass it back to your hands and lower your hands to the floor above your head.

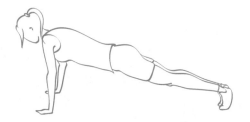

3. PLANK: This is basically holding the top of a pushup and keeping your body stiff like a plank. So start off lying face down, hands flat beneath your shoulders, push yourself up, then balance on your hands and toes.

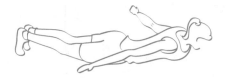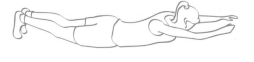

4. SUPERGIRL: Think superman flying, only cooler! Lie face down on the floor, lift up just your chest, arms, and legs, and extend your body as far as you can. For the **Supergirl Swimming** version of this exercise, do this same thing but move your arms as though you are doing a breaststroke in the water.

BEGINNER CORE	ADVANCED CORE
1. 10 BICYCLES	1. 20 BICYCLES
2. 10 V-UPS	2. 20 V-UPS
3. HOLD PLANK FOR 30 SECONDS	3. HOLD A PLANK FOR 60 SECONDS
4. HOLD SUPERGIRL FOR 30 SECONDS	4. HOLD SUPERGIRL SWIMMING FOR 30 SECONDS

Repeat these exercise sequences three times. If they are too hard, just do as many as you can, and work your way up.

Now that you know how to strengthen your core, let's move on to the rest of your body.

UPPER AND LOWER BODY STRENGTH EXERCISES

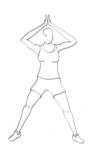

1. **JUMPING JACKS:** You probably know this. Jump up and down while spreading legs out to the side then back together, and alternate clapping your hands over your head and on your thighs.

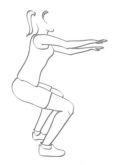

2. SQUATS: Stand tall, feet shoulder-width apart, knees slightly bent, arms up in front of you. Slowly squat down as if you're going to sit on a chair, then lift yourself back up to the original position.

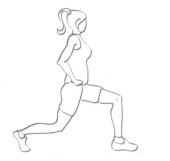 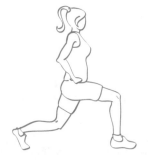

3. ALTERNATING LUNGES: Stand with hands on hips, put one foot about 3 feet in front of you while bending at both knees, then pull that same foot back next to the stationary foot. Then repeat move with the opposite foot.

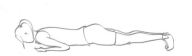 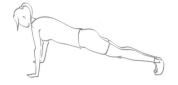 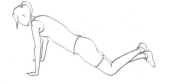

4. **PUSHUPS:** Lie face down on the floor, hands beneath your shoulders, push up off the floor to balance on toes and hands while keeping your body straight, then lower yourself part way by bending at the elbows. If it's too tough, try it with your knees on the floor instead of your toes.

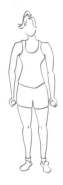 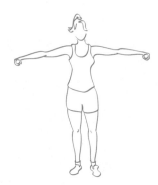

5. **LATERAL LIFTS:** Stand with your feet shoulder-width apart holding a light dumbell in each hand, with your arms hanging down along your sides. Slowly lift the weights out until your arms are parallel to the floor—like you're flying! Hold for a second, then slowly lower your arms back down and repeat.

UPPER AND LOWER BODY STRENGTH SEQUENCES

BEGINNER	ADVANCED
1. 25 JUMPING JACKS	1. 50 JUMPING JACKS
2. 10 SQUATS	2. 20 SQUATS
3. 10 ALTERNATING LUNGES	3. 10 ALTERNATING LUNGES (WHILE HOLDING 3 TO 5 POUNDS OF WEIGHT IN EACH HAND)
4. 10 PUSHUPS (ON KNEES)	4. 10 PUSHUPS (ON TOES)
5. 10 LATERAL LIFTS (WITH 2 TO 3 POUND WEIGHTS)	5. 10 LATERAL LIFTS (WITH 3 TO 5 POUND WEIGHTS)

Repeat these exercise sequences three times. If they are too hard, just do as many as you can and work your way up.

FLEXIBILITY: STRETCH BETTER!

Unhealthy body tissue is weak and tight. Healthy tissue is strong *and* elastic. Flexibility training is just as important as strength and cardio for overall fitness and for keeping your muscles working in peak condition. You might not be thinking about this now, but loss of flexibility is the first sign of aging; if you get and stay flexible now, you'll be in better shape for the rest of your life!

Flexibility training stretches should be held for at least 30 to 60 seconds to be effective. As you stretch, breathe deeply and be aware of the muscles you're using and how they're being lengthened.

STRETCHING SHOULD NOT HURT! If you can't hold a certain position for more than 30 seconds, you are probably trying to push too much at one time. Trust your body to tell you when you're straining too hard (it'll hurt!) and when you're doing it just right. (There will be some tension, but you'll feel your muscles start to give after several seconds.)

The following are some stretching exercises that you can do almost anywhere, even in front of the TV.

 Stretch like a cat when you wake up, even before you get out of bed.

 Sit on the floor with your legs straight out in a V, reach with your hands over your left leg for your left foot and hold; then reach straight out in front of you and hold; finally, reach for your right foot and hold. Stay in each position for at least 30 seconds.

 From a standing position, bend forward at the hips, hang your head down, and hold for about a minute.

 Roll your head slowly down toward your chest, then to your left shoulder, then back, then to your right shoulder, and back to your chest. Repeat 5 times.

☆ Reach your hands behind your back, interlace your fingers, straighten your arms, then lift the hands away from your lower back. Hold for 30 seconds.

☆ Reach arms over your head, interlace your fingers with your palms up, bend from your waist to the right, and hold for 30 seconds. Straighten back up and bend to the other side for 30 seconds.

EXERCISE BURNOUT

After you've exercised regularly for a while, you might experience exercise burnout. It's normal. At some point, almost everyone feels burned out or unmotivated to exercise. You also may get sick of the same old workout routine. If this happens, don't be afraid to try something new.

☆ **Exercise with a friend who can help push you to the next level.**

☆ **Go on a light jog and finish with a 50– or 100–yard dash to end your workout on a strong note and leave you feeling energized.**

☆ **Try kickboxing, yoga, bicycling, swimming, and hiking.**

☆ **Check out your local YMCA, which may have gyms, a pool, or offer classes and special rates for students.**

☆ Jump rope.

☆ Roll down a hill, hula hoop, roller skate—act like a little kid once in a while!

☆ Listen to music while you work out.

☆ Try aerobic chair dancing! Really! Check out www.chairdancing.com.

Be adventurous. Try all kinds of activities and find what you love. Bottom line: keep working on improving yourself and your level of fitness. Pay attention to even the smallest success—this will help push you to the next level!

Caution: There is such a thing as too much exercise. Two important things to know:

1. Your bone "growth plates" are open right now, meaning they're developing and still growing during your teen years. Overexercising can stop those growth plates from functioning properly and therefore stunt your growth! That's why we've kept this exercise program very basic. If you find that your body remains sore even after your initial few workouts—to the point where you can't walk and you ache all over—you'll know that you've gone too far.

OVERALL EXERCISE BENEFITS

♥ STRONGER BONES AND MUSCLES WILL ALLOW YOU TO EXERT MORE FORCE WITH MORE EASE, WHETHER YOU'RE LIFTING A BOOKBAG OR YOUR LITTLE BROTHER!

♥ MORE ENERGY WILL HELP YOU RUN FARTHER, DANCE LONGER, AND PLAY HARDER.

♥ FLEXIBILITY WILL KEEP YOU AGILE, YOUTHFUL, AND FEELING GREAT.

♥ INSTANT THERAPY IS WHAT A GREAT WORKOUT FEELS LIKE. YOU'LL FEEL CALM AND PEACEFUL, YET ENERGIZED.

♥ BETTER SLEEP IS ESPECIALLY IMPORTANT FOR TEENS, WHEN YOUR BODY'S CIRCADIAN RHYTHMS (AN INTERNAL BIOLOGICAL CLOCK) ARE RESET, TELLING YOU TO FALL ASLEEP LATER AND WAKE UP LATER. EXERCISE WILL HELP YOU FALL ASLEEP MORE EASILY AND WAKE UP MORE REFRESHED.

♥ A MORE ACTIVE SOCIAL LIFE WILL COME NATURALLY WHEN YOU EXERCISE AND PLAY SPORTS; YOU'LL MEET NEW PEOPLE, GAIN A SENSE OF ACCOMPLISHMENT, AND BOOST SELF-ESTEEM ALONG THE WAY.

2. If you're exercising a lot and not eating enough, your body won't be able to burn fat the way it should (i.e. you'll lower your metabolism and find it harder to lose weight). You really need to fuel your body with nutritious calories. This is not the time to deprive yourself of good food!

Sometimes many of us sabotage ourselves when we are dieting and working out. You know the excuses: I'm tired, it's late, etc. How do you motivate yourself? Have a little talk with yourself, and every time you have a negative thought, make it positive.

NEGATIVE SELF-TALK	POSITIVE SELF-TALK
"I JUST ATE A CANDY BAR. I NEED TO PUNISH MYSELF BY WORKING OUT."	"IT'S NOT THE END OF THE WORLD. I'LL FEEL BETTER IF I WORK OUT, BY RELEASING STRESS AND TENSION."
"I'M TOO FAT TO EXERCISE. IT WON'T MAKE A DIFFERENCE."	"OVER TIME, I KNOW IT WILL MAKE A DIFFERENCE. I'LL START WITH WALKING A LITTLE MORE, THEN GO FROM THERE."

"I'M JUST TOO LAZY TO WORK OUT."

"I CAN MAKE EXCUSES ALL DAY. WHAT I WANT IS CHANGE, AND TO KNOW WHAT IT FEELS LIKE TO LOVE MY BODY. ANY PHYSICAL ACTIVITY IS BETTER THAN NONE."

"I DON'T HAVE TIME TO WORK OUT."

"I DON'T HAVE TO RUN A MARATHON. I'LL JUST GO FOR A 20-MINUTE WALK OR JOG."

"EXERCISE DOESN'T WORK. I'VE TRIED IT."

"MY BODY AND MY HEALTH ARE IMPORTANT TO ME. THIS TIME, I'LL REALLY STICK TO AN EXERCISE PLAN UNTIL I SEE RESULTS."

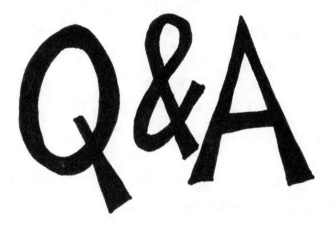

IS IT BETTER TO EXERCISE BEFORE OR AFTER A MEAL?

Eat first, then exercise. Most people don't realize that eating before you exercise will help your body burn calories more efficiently during your workout. Try eating a small amount of carbs and protein (like cheese and a few crackers) 1 to 2 hours before you exercise, so you'll be fueled up for your workout.

DOES EATING LOTS OF PROTEIN BUILD MUSCLE?

No. Although you need adequate protein to repair body tissues, eating *extra* protein does not boost muscle mass and strength. Eating more protein and increasing calories while maintaining your exercise level will only build an equal amount of additional fat and muscle mass. High-protein diets can dehydrate you as well as contribute to the loss of muscle and bone mass.

ONCE I'VE LOST ALL THE WEIGHT I WANT, DO I STILL NEED TO WORK OUT?

Absolutely! Once you've reached your goal weight, you'll want to maintain it. Keep working out at least 3 times a week. Recheck your BMI number from time to time. Stay active!

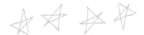

LACK OF ACTIVITY DESTROYS THE GOOD CONDITION OF EVERY HUMAN BEING, WHILE MOVEMENT AND METHODICAL PHYSICAL EXERCISE SAVE IT AND PRESERVE IT.

—PLATO

WHEN SHE'S GONE TOO FAR

TEN

ONE OUT OF EVERY SIX YOUNG WOMEN HAS "DISORDERED EATING" BEHAVIOR.

This is a tough chapter because eating disorders are a serious health issue, and people who have them are often in denial. Plus it's not easy recovering from disorders like bulimia, anorexia, and compulsive eating. You may have a friend who is in trouble, who's crossed the line between dieting and damaging. Perhaps you're wondering if you might have an eating disorder yourself. There's so much to learn about these issues. Read on!

An eating disorder isn't just an occasional binge, sporadically working out like crazy to burn calories, or skipping the occasional meal. It might start out like that, but a real eating disorder takes over your world and rules your life. The most common eating disorders among teenagers are:

 ANOREXIA **(starving yourself)**

 BULIMIA **(stuffing yourself then vomiting)**

 BINGE EATING **(compulsive eating, without vomiting)**

 USING LAXATIVES AND DIURETICS **(pills and diet aids that force your body to relieve itself)**

What many teenagers don't know is that these eating behaviors aren't even that effective. For example, vomiting does *not* get rid of all the food in your stomach; more than half the calories you eat during a binge get absorbed by your body. Laxatives and diuretics don't really stop calories from being absorbed—they just help you go to the bathroom and give you the false feeling that you're getting rid of calories when you're not. Very few young women know that these eating behaviors can be dangerous and even *deadly*.

Your teeth can rot from repeated exposure to the acid in vomit. Your stomach or throat can rip open from vomiting contractions. You can experience sudden seizures from chemical imbalances due to malnutrition. You can develop peptic ulcers. Your immune system weakens. Worst of all, you could literally starve yourself to death.

UP TO 20 PERCENT OF PEOPLE WITH SERIOUS EATING DISORDERS DIE IF UNTREATED.

PEOPLE WHO GET TREATMENT CAN FULLY RECOVER.

What causes an eating disorder? There's no clear-cut answer, but biological, social, and psychological factors all play a role. Low self-esteem, depression, a desire to be in control, society's relentless love affair with impossibly thin people—all of these things can be damaging to vulnerable souls.

Roughly 95 percent of teenagers with eating disorders are girls. Most of these girls juggle many different diets, constantly going on and off of them. Ironically, abusing otherwise healthy diets in this way can actually lead to eating disorders! Super strict diets leave people ravenous, and often cause them to overeat. When they overeat, they have a tendency to panic, and a vicious cycle begins.

Some people turn to these eating habits because of fear—fear of being fat, fear of losing control, fear of not being accepted, and so on. Bulimics and anorexics are often people who have little control of their lives and try to assert control by overmonitoring their food intake.

People with certain personality traits seem to be more vulnerable to eating disorders. Among them are people pleasers (good little girls) who've been raised to ignore their feelings and attend to the needs of others; perfectionists with low self-esteem; people who have a lot of general or social anxiety; people who've been teased about their body shape and weight; victims of sexual abuse; and people in dysfunctional families.

You can often tell if someone's in the grip of an eating disorder by watching out for the following signs:

ANOREXIA (STARVING YOURSELF)

☆ **Has drastic and sudden weight loss**

☆ **Maintains body weight way below normal**

☆ **Eats very little, plays with food**

☆ **Skips meals**

210

- Won't eat in front of other people
- Wears loose clothing to hide weight loss
- Exercises compulsively
- May stop having periods
- Says she's too fat when she's not
- Makes excuses not to eat

BULIMIA (STUFFING YOURSELF THEN VOMITING)

- Has frequent weight fluctuations
- Spends a lot of time in the bathroom, especially after meals
- Eats a lot without gaining significant weight
- Exercises obsessively to make up for overeating
- Has irregular or absent menstrual periods
- Uses laxatives

- Has damaged tooth enamel from vomiting

- Buys lots of food that suddenly disappears

- Has knuckles scraped from inducing vomiting

- Runs shower or sink to cover vomiting noises

- Vomits in the bathroom leaving it smelly

- Binges and purges more than two times a week

BINGE EATING
(COMPULSIVE EATING WITHOUT VOMITING)

- Feels "out of control" around food

- Is constantly planning food intake

- Eats in private

- Buys large amounts of food that disappears quickly

- Consumes vast quantities of food, usually at least over 2500 calories in one sitting

- Binges at least two times a week

USING LAxATIVES AND DIURETICS

 Goes to the bathroom often

 Purchases laxatives and diuretics often

There is also a disorder called BDD or Body Dysmorphic Disorder. It's not considered an official medical diagnosis, but it may achieve that status soon. BDD sufferers become obsessed with their body shape, size, weight, perceived lack of muscles, facial blemishes, and so forth, and they don't see themselves as they really are. About 70 percent of BDD cases begin before the age of eighteen.

FROM THE STRANGE BUT TRUE FILES

You may have heard of websites that are like secret clubs for anorexics and bulimics. They "teach" people how to starve themselves and vomit. To an outsider, it sounds bizarre, but people with these diseases find comfort and a sense of belonging at these websites. Chances are, they know nothing about nutrition and the damage they are causing their body.

These sites and chat rooms prey on the insecurities of young people, who are particularly vulnerable to peer pressure. In fact, after reading many online letters we found one that reflects a girl's awakening to the fact that these disorders don't really solve problems.

DEAR ANA [ANA=ANOREXIA],

I FEEL TRAPPED BY YOU . . . WHERE IS THE LOVE YOU PROMISED? THE ACCEPTANCE? WHEN WILL I FEEL LIKE I'M FINALLY IN CONTROL? WHY IS IT THAT THE MORE I CONTROL WHAT I EAT AND PURGE, THE MORE OUT OF CONTROL I FEEL?

—ANONYMOUS

Girls who are anorexic or bulimic often have distorted body images; they often think they're overweight when they're not, or fat when they're really too thin. They don't realize that restricting calories and mistreating their bodies will damage them in the long run, possibly stunting their growth and maybe even killing them.

If you know someone who may be a victim of one of these disorders, be as supportive as you can. Avoid talking about food. Let her know that you love her no matter how much or how little she weighs, but that you worry about her health. If she won't admit she has a problem, try to get help from an adult you can trust. You could also suggest a therapist. Or let her know about the following great websites, which will give her real information and offer real help:

- ☆ ANRED **(Anorexia Nervosa and Related Eating Disorders) www.anred.com**

- ☆ ANAD **(National Association of Anorexia Nervosa and Associated Disorders) www.anad.org**

- ☆ OVEREATERS ANONYMOUS **www.overeatersanonymous.org**

Bottom line: People with eating disorders have forgotten that eating should be a normal and healthy pleasure. You can't always eat perfectly. You won't always feel great about the way you eat. But starving yourself or putting yourself near death's door with an eating disorder is serious self-abuse. It takes a lot of wisdom and maturity to see that. Unfortunately, most people with eating disorders don't have those characteristics. Yet.

FICTION

FACT

IF YOU DIET AND EXERCISE LIKE CRAZY AND GET REALLY THIN, THEN PEOPLE WILL LIKE YOU A WHOLE LOT MORE.

PEOPLE LIKE EACH OTHER FOR LOTS OF REASONS. THEY REMAIN FRIENDS BECAUSE THEY LIKE EACH OTHER'S PERSONALITIES—NOT BECAUSE THEY ARE THIN.

215

FICTION	FACT
CELEBRITIES AND MODELS ARE SO LUCKY. I'LL NEVER BE ABLE TO LOOK LIKE THAT.	LISTEN, IF YOU HAD THE BEST MAKEUP ARTIST, STYLIST, PERSONAL TRAINER, AND EXPENSIVE BEAUTY PRODUCTS, YOU WOULD LOOK LIKE A CELEBRITY, TOO! AND REMEMBER, CELEBRITIES HAVE THEIR OWN STRUGGLES WITH EATING DISORDERS.
TO LOSE WEIGHT, YOU SHOULD NEVER EAT FATTY FOODS, SWEETS, OR DESSERTS.	DEPRIVING YOURSELF OF THE FOODS YOU LOVE WILL ONLY BACKFIRE AND MAKE YOU UNHAPPY. EAT SOME OF WHAT YOU LOVE SOME OF THE TIME. ENJOY! JUST DON'T GO CRAZY.
THOSE HUNGER PANGS ARE A GOOD SIGN; THEY MEAN YOU'RE LOSING WEIGHT.	NOPE, HUNGER PANGS MEAN YOUR BODY NEEDS FUEL. IF YOU LET YOURSELF GO HUNGRY FOR LONG PERIODS OF TIME, YOUR METABOLISM SLOWS DOWN AND IT'S HARDER TO BURN FAT WHEN YOU DO START EATING AGAIN. LISTEN TO THOSE HUNGER PANGS!

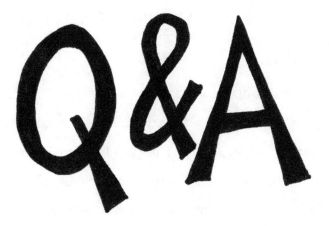

Q&A

I THINK I MAY HAVE AN EATING DISORDER, BUT I DON'T KNOW WHERE TO TURN, AND I'M NOT READY TO TALK TO ANYONE ABOUT IT. WHAT SHOULD I DO?

You've made a good decision by even admitting that. Go hang out at a bookstore and start browsing through the self-help section for books on eating disorders. Then check out the websites listed in this chapter. Start gathering information. When you're brave enough, and when you realize that your health and long life are more important to you than your eating disorder, get help. The websites listed on page 215 provide phone numbers of help hotlines that will respect your privacy.

I'VE BEEN USING LAXATIVES AND ENEMAS TO CONTROL MY WEIGHT. AFTER I USE THEM, I ALWAYS WEIGH LESS THAN I DID BEFORE. WHAT'S WRONG WITH THAT?

Don't fool yourself. Laxatives and enemas remove lots of *water* from the colon—not just food residue—which can cause severe dehydration. The minute you start drinking liquids again, the weight will return. Laxatives and enemas remove neither fat nor calories, since your food has already passed through your stomach and been absorbed. All you're doing is getting rid of body waste.

You should also know that enemas can stretch out the colon, leaving it limp with no muscle tone. When this happens, the muscles can't contract and move fecal matter out of the body.

I TRY NOT TO BINGE AND PURGE, BUT WHEN I SEE ALL THESE THIN PEOPLE IN MAGAZINES AND ON TV, AND EVEN OTHER GIRLS IN MY SCHOOL WHO LOOK SO HAPPY, I JUST WANT TO BE THIN SO BADLY.

If you want to be thin, work at it, but do it the right way. Don't abuse yourself. The media is a powerful force. But remember, it's not reality.

Here's an interesting story. In 1995, before television came to the island of Fiji, people thought the ideal body was round and soft and plump. After three years of TV shows like *Melrose Place, Beverly Hills 90210,* and other slick shows, Fijian teenagers started showing serious signs of eating disorders. So remember the destructive force of these media images the next time they flash in front of you.

I CAN'T AFFORD A THERAPIST OR SPECIAL PROGRAMS TO HELP ME STOP. WHERE CAN I FIND AFFORDABLE HELP?

Go on the Internet and visit the chat rooms of websites such as www.anad.org or www.overeatersanonymous.com. Read everything you can. Start confiding in friends and telling them what's going on with you. Write e-mails to the sites and call their hotlines; they'll be able to steer you toward help.

ABOVE ALL, TAKE CARE OF YOURSELF!

You are more than just a body. You are a living, breathing soul with emotions and feelings. When the urge to abuse yourself takes hold, pause.

Take your hand and hold your own cheek, like a loving parent would do. Feel the calm. Go to a mirror and pat yourself on the back. Tell yourself you're going to be okay. For at least this one brief moment, be good to yourself.

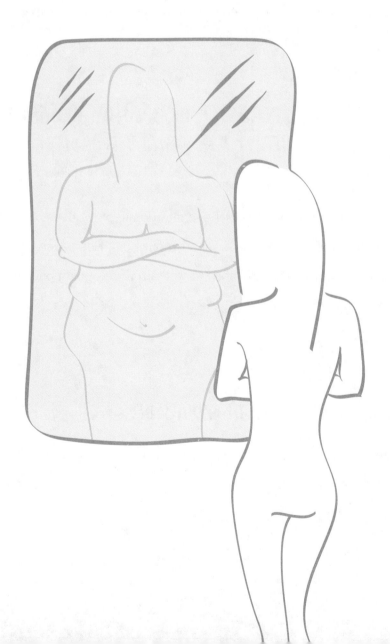

P. S. !

We have just a few things left to give you:

1. **Your Food Diary**

2. **Measuring for Success**

3. **The Best Diet Tips Ever**

YOUR FOOD DIARY

A food diary can really make a difference. In fact, statistics show that people who use a food diary *and* a meal plan lose more weight than people who don't. We've included a 7-day diary here, but feel free to make extra copies if you need more.

Here's how to use it. Keep track of everything you eat in a 24-hour period, then compare it with your meal plan and calorie goals. Doing this on a daily basis will help you stay on track! We promise! Just make sure you're honest with yourself. (No one else is supposed to see your food diary anyway.) Write down:

⭐ **Everything you eat (even if it's licking the cookie dough spoon)**

⭐ **Everything you do (like stretching, working out, running, playing sports, etc.)**

⭐ **How you feel (note your feelings throughout the day—such as tired, hungry, sleepy, energetic, etc.)**

Also jot down extra details like how much you slept the night before and how you feel when you wake up. It's also good to keep track of your emotions. You'll be surprised at what you learn about yourself!

MY FOOD DIARY

DATE	AMOUNT	CALORIES
BREAKFAST		
LUNCH		
DINNER		
SNACKS		

MY MOOD TODAY	NOTES

GLASSES OF WATER I DRANK TODAY

P.S.!

MY FOOD DIARY

DATE		AMOUNT	CALORIES
BREAKFAST			
LUNCH			
DINNER			
SNACKS			

MY MOOD TODAY	NOTES

GLASSES OF WATER I DRANK TODAY

224

MY FOOD DIARY

DATE	AMOUNT	CALORIES
BREAKFAST		
LUNCH		
DINNER		
SNACKS		

MY MOOD TODAY	NOTES

GLASSES OF WATER I DRANK TODAY

MY FOOD DIARY

DATE		AMOUNT	CALORIES
BREAKFAST			
LUNCH			
DINNER			
SNACKS			

MY MOOD TODAY	NOTES

GLASSES OF WATER I DRANK TODAY

MY FOOD DIARY

DATE		AMOUNT	CALORIES
BREAKFAST			
LUNCH			
DINNER			
SNACKS			

MY MOOD TODAY	NOTES

GLASSES OF WATER I DRANK TODAY

P.S.!

MY FOOD DIARY

DATE		AMOUNT	CALORIES
BREAKFAST			
LUNCH			
DINNER			
SNACKS			

MY MOOD TODAY	NOTES

GLASSES OF WATER I DRANK TODAY

228

MY FOOD DIARY

DATE		AMOUNT	CALORIES
BREAKFAST			
LUNCH			
DINNER			
SNACKS			

MY MOOD TODAY	NOTES

GLASSES OF WATER I DRANK TODAY

MEASURING FOR SUCCESS

	MONTH 1	MONTH 2	MONTH 3	MONTH 4
CHEST (AT WIDEST POINT)				
BICEP (UPPER ARM, AT WIDEST POINT)				
WAIST (½" ABOVE BELLY BUTTON)				
HIPS (STAND WITH FEET TOGETHER AND MEASURE AT WIDEST POINT OF BUTTOCKS)				
BMI #				

THE BEST DIET TIPS EVER

♥ Going to Jamba Juice or Robeks-type place? Ask for a kid-size drink! Or split a regular-size one with a friend.

♥ Ask for half the normal serving of vanilla or chocolate powder/syrup in drinks at Starbucks or other coffee shops.

♥ Dilute apple juice with water or add lots of ice.

♥ Feel a binge coming on? Go gargle with mouthwash and wait 15 minutes. The urge to eat will most likely go away.

♥ Put a cute sign on your refrigerator that says, "Are you looking in here because you're bored?"

♥ Call yourself on the phone and leave a message saying you are proud of yourself and to keep up the good work.

♥ Hang your swimsuit on the refrigerator.

♥ Avoid drinking soda.

♥ Always, always eat breakfast.

♥ Remember, your next meal is more important than your last one.

♥ Make your meals smaller as the day goes by.

♥ Don't eat big meals at the end of the day.

♥ Try to stop eating by 8:00 P.M.

OH YEAH, ONE MORE THING . . .

YOU MIGHT WANT TO CHECK OUT THESE GREAT WEBSITES:

www.hungry-girl.com Tips and tricks for hungry chicks!

www.blubberbusters.com A website about being overweight.

www.girlsinc.org A website that encourages girls to be strong, smart, and bold.

www.kidshealth.org Full of information about all aspects of health.

www.cdc.gov/powerfulbones A website for young teenagers filled with fun ways to recognize the importance of strong bones.

www.fda.gov (click on "Teens" under the "Information For" list) A website filled with information on current health issues.

www.chairdancing.com A fun aerobic workout you can do while sitting in a chair—great for those who are really overweight!

www.geneenroth.com Soothing and wise website for people with eating disorders.

AFTERWORD

HEY SAVVY GIRL,

So there you have it—all the information, nutrition, and love we could possibly give you so that you won't have to ride a diet merry-go-round for the rest of your life. We want you to have a healthy relationship with food. It's not your enemy. If you learn that now, while you're young, your life will be a lot sweeter.

We want you to be good to yourself. We want you to be fit, healthy, and nutritionally smart. Remember to tune in to your body's messages. Pay attention to when you're really hungry, and stop eating when you're satisfied (not stuffed). Get familiar with that pleasantly full feeling and enjoy it. When you make good food choices, you're taking care of yourself!

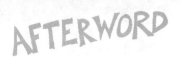

Most of all, we want you to live with passion and joy and self-confidence. You deserve to feel beautiful inside and out. You deserve to go after your dreams. This is your life. Make it a great one!

Love,

Carrie and Barbara

 HELLO WORLD, THIS IS ME.

—BELLE PEREZ, FROM THE SONG "HELLO WORLD"

ACKNOWLEDGMENTS

Thanks to my precious daughter, Bella, and to the rest of my family, Mom, Dad, Peter, Andi, Stu, Spencer, and Haley. You are all the joy, the love, and the foundation of my life. To my dedicated team at Diet Designs, Mario, Rachel, and Beth, you are all the best! To Jamie Zamhad, thank you for your contribution to this book. To Barbara, thank you for your commitment, endless energy, and total love you poured into this book. To my publisher, Judith Regan, thank you for your passion in disseminating information and giving people the tools to change their lives. To my amazing editor, Anna Bliss, it was a pleasure to work with you.

To all my young readers, savor this time in your life, do your best to reach your full potential—physically, spiritually, intellectually—and, most of all, enjoy the process!

—Carrie Wiatt

235

ACKNOWLEDGMENTS

I would like to give a big thanks to Judith Regan for taking the call and for being the kind of woman others can learn from. To Anna Bliss, thanks for your patience and for making this book better. A big thank you to Carrie for her expertise, knowledge, and dedication to this project. To my incredible daughter Glenn, who is the best secret weapon a mom could have when it comes to editing a book like this. You amaze and inspire me. A big thanks to all the girls in our surveys and focus groups, especially Julia Roth, Zoe Worth, and my niece Libby, you're all gems! To my son Gage for *trying* to eat a healthier diet. And finally to my extraordinary husband Richard, for keeping the junk food in the house on the left side of the pantry.

—Barbara Schroeder

BIBLIOGRAPHY

Piper, Mary Bray. *Hunger Pains.* New York: Ballantine Books, 1997.

Richardson, Brenda Lane and Elane Rehr. *101 Ways to Help Your Daughter Love Her Body*. New York: Quill, 2001.

Schwartz, Erika. *The Teen Weight-Loss Solution.* New York: William Morrow, 2004.

WEBSITES

www.anad.org

www.anred.com

www.blubberbusters.com

www.cdc.gov/powerfulbones

www.chairdancing.com

www.fda.gov

www.fda.com

www.geneenroth.com

BIBLIOGRAPHY

www.girlsinc.org

www.hungry-girl.com

www.intelihealth.com

www.kidshealth.com

www.llu.edu

www.nih.gov

www.overeatersanonymous.org

www.webmd.com

STUDIES AND SURVEYS

American Academy of Pediatrics general policy statement.

Centers for Disease Control and Prevention National Survey, 2002.

Harvard Medical School Teen Survey. Anne Becker, director of research Harvard Eating Disorders Center, 1998.

Journal of the American Dietetic Association's Teen Dieting Survey. Laura Calderon PhD, RD, 2004.

National Health and Nutrition Examination Survey, 1999–2000.

"A Pavlovian Approach to the Problem of Obesity" *International Journal of Obesity*, July 2004.

"The Surgeon General's Call to Action to Prevent and Decrease Overweight and Obesity" 2001.

"Teen Obesity" *Health Journal of Epidemiology*. Dr. Anders Engelend, Norwegian Institute of Public Health, January 2004.

INDEX

INDEX

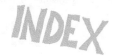

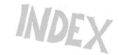

INDEX